Orofacial Pain

Editors

SCOTT S. DE ROSSI
DAVID A. SIROIS

DENTAL CLINICS OF NORTH AMERICA

www.dental.theclinics.com

July 2013 • Volume 57 • Number 3

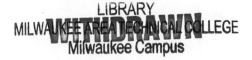

ELSEVIER

1600 John F. Kennedy Boulevard • Suite 1800 • Philadelphia, Pennsylvania, 19103-2899

http://www.dental.theclinics.com

DENTAL CLINICS OF NORTH AMERICA Volume 57, Number 3
July 2013 ISSN 0011-8532, ISBN 978-1-4557-5635-3

Editor: Yonah Korngold; y.korngold@elsevier.com

Dental Clinics of North America (ISSN 0011-8532) is published quarterly by Elsevier Inc., 360 Park Avenue South, New York, NY 10010-1710. Months of issue are January, April, July, and October. Business and Editorial Offices: 1600 John F. Kennedy Boulevard, Suite 1800, Philadelphia, PA 19103-2899. Periodicals postage paid at New York, NY and additional mailing offices. Subscription prices are $269.00 per year (domestic individuals), $474.00 per year (domestic institutions), $127.00 per year (domestic students/residents), $322.00 per year (Canadian individuals), $595.00 per year (Canadian institutions), $390.00 per year (international individuals), $595.00 per year (international institutions), and $192.00 per year (international and Canadian students/residents). International air speed delivery is included in all *Clinics* subscription prices. All prices are subject to change without notice. **POSTMASTER:** Send address changes to *Dental Clinics of North America*, Elsevier Health Sciences Division, Subscription Customer Service, 3251 Riverport Lane, Maryland Heights, MO 63043. **Customer Service (orders, claims, online, change of address): Elsevier Health Sciences Division, Subscription Customer Service, 3251 Riverport Lane, Maryland Heights, MO 63043. Tel: 1-800-654-2452 (U.S. and Canada). Fax: 314-447-8029. E-mail: journalscustomer service-usa@elsevier.com (for print support); journalsonlinesupport-usa@elsevier.com (for online support).**

Reprints. For copies of 100 or more, of articles in this publication, please contact the Commercial Reprints Department, Elsevier Inc., 360 Park Avenue South, New York, NY 10010-1710. Tel.: 212-633-3812; Fax: 212-462-1935; E-mail: reprints@elsevier.com.

The *Dental Clinics of North America* is covered in *MEDLINE/PubMed (Index Medicus), Current Contents/Clinical Medicine, ISI/BIOMED* and *Clinahl.*

Printed in the United States of America.

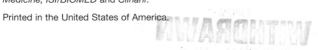

Contributors

EDITORS

SCOTT S. DE ROSSI, DMD
Chair, Department of Oral Health and Diagnostic Sciences, College of Dental Medicine; Associate Professor, Departments of Dermatology and Otolaryngology/Head and Neck Surgery, Medical College of Georgia, Georgia Regents University, Augusta, Georgia

DAVID A. SIROIS, DMD, PhD
Oral and Maxillofacial Pathology, Radiology and Medicine, New York University College of Dentistry; Department of Neurology, New York University School of Medicine, New York, New York

AUTHORS

RAFAEL BENOLIEL, BDS, LDS RCS ENG
Professor, Department of Oral Medicine, The Faculty of Dentistry, Hebrew University-Hadassah, Jerusalem, Israel

MICHAEL T. BRENNAN, DDS, MHS
Department of Oral Medicine, Carolinas Medical Center, Charlotte, North Carolina

KATHARINE N. CIARROCCA, DMD, MSEd
Assistant Professor, Department of Oral Rehabilitation; Division of Geriatric Dentistry, Deparment of Oral Health and Diagnostic Sciences, College of Dental Medicine, Georgia Regents University, Augusta, Georgia

SCOTT S. DE ROSSI, DMD
Chairman, Department of Oral Health and Diagnostic Sciences, College of Dental Medicine; Associate Professor, Departments of Dermatology and Otolaryngology/Head and Neck Surgery, Medical College of Georgia, Georgia Regents University, Augusta, Georgia

ELI ELIAV, DMD, PhD
Professor, Robert and Susan Carmel Endowed Chair in Algesiology, Director, Division of Orofacial Pain, Chair, Department of Diagnostic Sciences, UMDNJ-New Jersey Dental School, Newark, New Jersey

F. JOHN FIRRIOLO, DDS, PhD
Professor of Oral Medicine, Department of General Dentistry and Oral Medicine, School of Dentistry, University of Louisville, Louisville, Kentucky

MARTIN S. GREENBERG, DDS, FDS RCS
Professor Oral Medicine, Department of Oral Medicine, Associate Dean Hospital Affairs, School of Dental Medicine, University of Pennsylvania, Philadelphia, Pennsylvania

GARY M. HEIR, DMD
Clinical Professor, Clinical Director, Center for Temporomandibular Disorders and Orofacial Pain, Department of Diagnostic Sciences, University of Medicine and Dentistry of New Jersey, New Jersey

ALLISON HUNTER, DMD, MS
Assistant Professor of Radiology, Department of Oral Health and Diagnostic Sciences, College of Dental Medicine, Georgia Regents University, Augusta, Georgia

WENDY S. HUPP, DMD
Associate Professor of Oral Medicine, Department of General Dentistry and Oral Medicine, School of Dentistry, University of Louisville, Louisville, Kentucky

SAJITHA KALATHINGAL, BDS, MS
Associate Professor of Radiology, Department of Oral Health and Diagnostic Sciences, College of Dental Medicine, Georgia Regents University, Augusta, Georgia

JUNAD KHAN, BDS, MSD, MPH, DAAOP
Assistant Professor, Department of Diagnostic Sciences, Center for Temporomandibular Disorders and Orofacial Pain, University of Medicine and Dentistry of New Jersey, New Jersey

ANIL KUMAR, DMD
Oral Medicine Resident, Department of Oral Medicine, Carolinas Medical Center, Charlotte, North Carolina

FREDERICK LIU, DDS, MD
Department of Oral and Maxillofacial Surgery, School of Dental Medicine, University of Pennsylvania, Philadelphia, Pennsylvania

JOEL J. NAPEÑAS, DDS
Assistant Professor, Division of Oral Medicine and Radiology, Schulich School of Medicine and Dentistry, Western University, London, Ontario, Canada; Department of Oral Medicine, Carolinas Medical Center, Charlotte, North Carolina

CIBELE NASRI-HEIR, DDS, MSD
Research Associate, Center for Temporomandibular Disorders and Orofacial Pain, Department of Diagnostic Sciences, University of Medicine and Dentistry of New Jersey, New Jersey

THOMAS P. SOLLECITO, DMD
Professor and Chairman of Oral Medicine, University of Pennsylvania School of Dental Medicine, Philadelphia, Pennsylvania

ANDREW STEINKELER, DMD, MD
Department of Oral and Maxillofacial Surgery, School of Dental Medicine, University of Pennsylvania, Philadelphia, Pennsylvania

ILANIT STERN, DMD
Clinical Instructor, Department of Oral Health and Diagnostic Sciences, Center for Oral Medicine, College of Dental Medicine, Georgia Regents University, Augusta, Georgia

JAISRI R. THOPPAY, BDS, MBA
Student, College of Graduate Studies, Georgia Regents University, Augusta, Georgia

Contents

Orofacial Pain: A Primer   383

Scott S. De Rossi

> Orofacial pain refers to pain associated with the soft and hard tissues of
> the head, face, and neck. It is a common experience in the population
> that has profound sociologic effects and impact on quality of life. New
> scientific evidence is constantly providing insight into the cause and
> pathophysiology of orofacial pain including temporomandibular disor-
> ders, cranial neuralgias, persistent idiopathic facial pains, headache,
> and dental pain. An evidence-based approach to the management of
> orofacial pain is imperative for the general clinician. This article reviews
> the basics of pain epidemiology and neurophysiology and sets the stage
> for in-depth discussions of various painful conditions of the head and
> neck.

**Clinical Assessment of Patients with Orofacial Pain and Temporomandibular
Disorders**   393

Ilanit Stern and Martin S. Greenberg

> Accurate diagnosis of chronic pain disorders of the mouth, jaws, and face
> is frequently complex. It is common for patients with chronic orofacial pain
> to consult multiple clinicians and receive ineffective treatment before a cor-
> rect diagnosis is reached. This problem is a significant public health con-
> cern. Clinicians can minimize error by starting the diagnostic procedure
> with a careful, accurate history and thorough head and neck examination
> followed by a thoughtfully constructed differential diagnosis. The possibil-
> ity that the patient has symptoms of a life-threatening underlying disease
> rather than a more common dental, sinus, or temporomandibular disorder
> must always be considered.

Diagnostic Imaging for Temporomandibular Disorders and Orofacial Pain   405

Allison Hunter and Sajitha Kalathingal

> The focus of this article is diagnostic imaging used for the evaluation of
> temporomandibular disorders and orofacial pain patients. Imaging modal-
> ities discussed include conventional panoramic radiography, panoramic
> temporomandibular joint imaging mode, cone beam computed tomogra-
> phy, and magnetic resonance imaging. The imaging findings associated
> with common diseases of the temporomandibular joint are presented
> and indications for brain imaging are discussed. Advantages and

disadvantages of each imaging modality are presented as well as illustrations of the various imaging techniques.

When a patient complains of orofacial pain, health care providers must make a correct diagnosis. Doing this can be difficult, since various signs and symptoms may not be specific for 1 particular problem or disorder. One initially should formulate a broad differential diagnosis that can be narrowed after analysis of the history and examination. In this article, orofacial pain is categorized as being caused by: intracranial pain, headaches, neuropathic pain, intraoral pain, temporomandibular disorder, cervical pain, pain related to anatomically associated structures, referred pain, or mental illness.

Dental and oral diseases are common findings in the general population. Pain associated with dental or periodontal disease is the primary reason why most patients seek treatment from providers. Thus, it is essential that all complaints of pain in the mouth and face include ruling out pain of dental origin. However, intraoral pain is not exclusively a result of dental disorders. This review outlines common somatic intraoral pain disorders, which can originate from disease involving one or more broad anatomic areas: the teeth, the surrounding soft tissues (mucogingival, tongue, and salivary glands), and bone.

Muscle disorders involving the masticatory muscles have been considered analogous to skeletal muscle disorders throughout the body. However, emerging research has shed new light on the varied etiology, clinical presentation, diagnosis, and treatment of myofascial pain and masticatory muscle disorders. This article reviews the etiology and classification of regional masticatory muscle disorders, the clinical examination of the patient, and evidence-based treatment recommendations.

Temporomandibular disorder (TMD) is a multifactorial disease process caused by muscle hyperfunction or parafunction, traumatic injuries, hormonal influences, and articular changes. Symptoms of TMD include decreased mandibular range of motion, muscle and joint pain, joint crepitus, and functional limitation or deviation of jaw opening. Only after failure of noninvasive options should more invasive and nonreversible treatments be initiated. Treatment can be divided into noninvasive, minimally invasive, and invasive options. Temporomandibular joint replacement is reserved for severely damaged joints with end-stage disease that has failed all other more conservative treatment modalities.

DENTAL CLINICS OF NORTH AMERICA

Erratum

An Error was made in the April 2013 issue of Dental Clinics on page 195 in the article "Oral Health and Dental Care During Pregnancy." The author Dr Hiroko Iida's last name was misspelled. Iida is the correct spelling.

Dent Clin N Am 57 (2013) ix
http://dx.doi.org/10.1016/j.cden.2013.06.001
0011-8532/13/$ – see front matter © 2013 Elsevier Inc. All rights reserved.

Preface

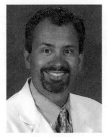 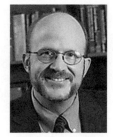

Scott S. De Rossi, DMD   David A. Sirois, DMD, PhD
Editors

Pain of the oral and maxillofacial structures encompasses aspects of general dental practice as well as medical and dental specialties. Pain has been considered a "fifth vital sign" and is a common presenting complaint among dental patients. Orofacial pain is a too prevalent and often debilitating condition with significant economic and social sequelae. In fact, the World Health Organization underscores the importance of pain and defines "oral health" as a "state of being free from chronic mouth and facial pain..." Oral health care providers are often involved in the prevention, evaluation, diagnosis, treatment, and rehabilitation of orofacial pain disorders. These disorders may have pain and associated symptoms arising from a discrete identifiable cause, such as postoperative pain or pain associated with a malignancy, or may be part of syndromes in which pain constitutes the primary problem, such as temporomandibular disorder pain, neuropathic pain, or headaches. The diagnosis of orofacial pain relies on interpretation of historical data; review of laboratory studies, imaging, behavioral, social, and occupational assessments; interview and examination by the clinician. Appropriate treatment of patients is dependent on an astute, knowledgeable, and dedicated clinician able to synthesize information from history and comprehensive clinical examination, to develop an accurate diagnosis, and to implement a treatment plan consistent with the standards of care based on currently available scientific literature.

This issue of *Dental Clinics of North America* combines the contributions of numerous world renowned clinical, research, and teaching scholars. And it has been a distinct pleasure to have assembled and worked with such an esteemed group. This work is not intended to be an all-encompassing text on all aspects of orofacial pain. Instead, it is a guide for clinicians in the care of their patients by providing evidence-based insight regarding patient assessment, diagnosis, and management.

I would like to acknowledge and thank my teachers, colleagues, residents, students, and patients, who have been a part of my career. For their loving support and instilling in me the desire to be an educator, I thank my parents, Steven and Catherine

Dent Clin N Am 57 (2013) xi–xii
http://dx.doi.org/10.1016/j.cden.2013.05.001
0011-8532/13/$ – see front matter © 2013 Published by Elsevier Inc.

dental.theclinics.com

De Rossi; and my wife, Dr Katharine Ciarrocca, and my daughters, Sofia and Evangelia, whose love, support, patience, and understanding have allowed me so many blessings.

Scott S. De Rossi, DMD
Department of Oral Health and Diagnostic Sciences
College of Dental Medicine
Department of Otolaryngology/Head & Neck Surgery
and Department of Dermatology
Medical College of Georgia
Georgia Regents University
1120 15th Street
Augusta, GA 30912, USA

David A. Sirois, DMD, PhD
Oral and Maxillofacial Pathology, Radiology and Medicine
New York University College of Dentistry
Department of Neurology
New York University School of Medicine
380 2nd Avenue, Suite 301
New York, NY 10010, USA

E-mail addresses:
SDEROSSI@gru.edu (S.S. De Rossi)
ds62@nyu.edu (D.A. Sirois)

Orofacial Pain: A Primer

Scott S. De Rossi, DMD[a,b,c,*]

KEYWORDS

- Orofacial pain • Myofascial pain • Temporomandibular disorder

KEY POINTS

- Orofacial pain refers to pain associated with the soft and hard tissues of the head, face, and neck. It is a common experience in the population that has profound sociologic effects and impact on quality of life.
- New scientific evidence is constantly providing insight into the cause and pathophysiology of orofacial pain including temporomandibular disorders, cranial neuralgias, persistent idiopathic facial pains, headache, and dental pain.
- An evidence-based approach to the management of orofacial pain is imperative for the general clinician.

INTRODUCTION

Orofacial pain refers to pain associated with the soft and hard tissues of the head, face, and neck. The potential origin of orofacial pain includes pulpal and periodontal, vascular, gland, muscle, bones, sinuses, and joint structures. These numerous structures in the head and neck along with their complex innervation account for the wide range of diagnostic possibilities in patients with the complaint of orofacial pain. The diverse potential for pain arising from the vast area of trigeminal innervation accounts for the need for interdisciplinary collaboration in the evaluation and treatment of these complex patients. Orofacial pain is a common experience in the population that has profound sociologic effects and impact on quality of life. It is estimated that one-third of the population of industrialized nations suffers some chronic pain and the oral health care provider will undoubtedly treat patients with orofacial pain. The cost of chronic pain is in the billions of dollars annually in the United States for health care services, loss of work, decreased productivity, and disability compensation. New scientific evidence is constantly providing insight into the cause and pathophysiology of orofacial pain. An evidence-based approach to the management of orofacial pain is imperative for the general clinician.

[a] Department of Oral health and Diagnostic Sciences, College of Dental Medicine, Georgia Regents University, 1120 15th Street, Augusta, GA 30912, USA; [b] Department of Otolaryngology/Head & Neck Surgery, Medical College of Georgia, Georgia Regents University, 1120 15th Street, Augusta, GA 30912, USA; [c] Department of Dermatology, Medical College of Georgia, Georgia Regents University, 1120 15th Street, Augusta, GA 30912, USA
* Department of Oral health and Diagnostic Sciences, College of Dental Medicine, Georgia Regents University, 1120 15th Street, Augusta, GA 30912, USA.
E-mail address: sderossi@gru.edu

Dent Clin N Am 57 (2013) 383–392
http://dx.doi.org/10.1016/j.cden.2013.04.001
0011-8532/13/$ – see front matter © 2013 Elsevier Inc. All rights reserved.

dental.theclinics.com

PROFESSIONAL RESPONSIBILITY

Pain in the oral and maxillofacial system represents a major medical and social problem in the United States. The US Surgeon General's report on Oral Health in America noted that oral health means more than healthy teeth; it means being free of chronic orofacial pain conditions (http://www.nidcr.nih.gov/DataStatistics/SurgeonGeneral/Report/ExecutiveSummary.htm).

The astute clinician possesses a working knowledge of the basic and clinical science of orofacial pain. To effectively evaluate and treat these patients, the clinician needs to ask questions, analyze answers, further question the patient, and synthesize information. The clinician must perform a proper clinical assessment including a comprehensive head and neck and dental physical examination, neurologic testing, range of motion studies, laboratory evaluation, and perhaps consultations with other health care providers. In addition, the clinician must develop a plan of treatment that is consistent with the standard of care set forth by current scientific literature and evidence. When the scope of care falls beyond the individual expertise of a clinician a team approach should be used and the patient should be referred.

Orofacial pain may be derived from many unique tissues of the head and neck, and subsequently has several unique physiologic characteristics compared with other pain systems, such as back or spinal pain. It is not surprising that accurate diagnosis and effective management of orofacial pain conditions represents a significant challenge for health care providers. Yet, this is an emerging and ever-growing area of dental practice. According to Hargreaves,[1] publications in the field of orofacial pain have demonstrated a steady increase over the last several decades. Robert and colleagues[2,3] published a bibliometric analysis of the scientific literature on pain research that was published in 2008. This paper demonstrated how complex the literature on orofacial pain is, indicating that 975 articles on orofacial pain were published in 275 journals from authors representing 54 countries. One of the biggest barriers for improved patient care and translational research has been the lack of a validated diagnostic criteria and varying terminologies between major groups that study pain.[1] Although efforts have been made to classify patients with temporomandibular disorders with research diagnostic criteria for temporomandibular disorders,[4] headache patients with the International Headache Society criteria, and orofacial pain with the American Academy of Orofacial Pain standards, clinical research suggests that these methods are incomplete for comprehensive diagnosis of patients with orofacial pain.[5,6] It is clear that translational research is necessary to ultimately improve diagnosis and patient care in patients with orofacial pain (**Table 1**).

EPIDEMIOLOGY OF OROFACIAL PAIN

Numerous reports in the scientific literature have attempted to identify the epidemiology of orofacial pain. The 1986 Nuprin Pain Report noted that most Americans experience an average of three or four different kinds of pain annually.[7] Crook and coworkers[8] reported that 16% of the general population suffered pain within a 2-week period. James and colleagues[9] in 1991 reported that greater than 81% of the population reported a significant jaw pain experience over the course of their lifetime. Lipton and coworkers[10] in 1993 noted that 22% of Americans reported orofacial pain within a 6-month period. Although the orofacial pain most commonly experienced by patients and encountered by oral health care providers is toothache, orofacial pain seldom seems to be an isolated complaint.[11] Türp and colleagues[12] noted that more than 81% of patients reporting to an orofacial pain center had pain sources beyond the trigeminal system. Common comorbid conditions include fibromyalgia, chronic

Table 1
Classification of pain: scheme for coding chronic pain diagnoses[a]

Axis	Definition
1	Regions (eg, head, face, and mouth)
2	Systems (eg, nervous system)
3	Temporal characteristics of pain (eg, continuous, recurring irregularly, paroxysmal)
4	Patient's statement of intensity: time since onset of pain (eg, mild, medium, severe; $\leq$1 mo; >6 mo)
5	Etiology (eg, genetic, infective, psychological)

[a] International Association for the Study of Pain classification.

fatigue syndrome, headache, panic disorder, gastroesophageal reflux disorder, irritable bowel syndrome, multiple chemical sensitivities, and posttraumatic stress disorder.[13] Often, symptoms for comorbid conditions may differentiate the patient with orofacial pain from patients seeking routine dental care or those with emergent or acute dental pain.[14] It is important that the clinician and the patient work to reveal all pain sources to improve prognosis and ensure appropriate therapy (**Table 2**).[12]

DEFINING PAIN

Orofacial pain is the presenting symptom of a broad spectrum of diseases. Pain is also interdisciplinary. Causes of orofacial pain may include diseases of orofacial structures; psychological abnormalities; referred pain from other sources, such as cervical muscles or intracranial pathology; and often most challenging for the clinician, orofacial pain may occur in the absence of detectable physical, imaging, or laboratory abnormalities.[15] The International Association for the Study of Pain defines pain as an unpleasant sensory and emotional experience associated with actual or potential tissue damage, or described in terms of such damage. Inherent in this definition is

Table 2
Differential diagnosis of orofacial pain[a]

Intracranial pain disorders	Neoplasm, aneurysm, abscess, hemorrhage, hematoma, edema
Primary headache disorders (neurovascular disorders)	Migraine, migraine variants, cluster headache, paroxysmal hemicrania, cranial arteritis Carotodynia, tension-type headache
Neurogenic pain disorders	Paroxysmal neuralgias (trigeminal, glossopharyngeal, nervus intermedius, superior laryngeal) Continuous pain disorders (deafferentation, neuritis, postherpetic neuralgia, posttraumatic and postsurgical neuralgia) Sympathetically maintained pain
Intraoral pain disorders	Dental pulp, periodontium, mucogingival tissues, tongue
Temporomandibular disorders	Masticatory muscle, temporomandibular joint, associated structures
Associated structures	Ears, eyes, nose, paranasal sinuses, throat, lymph nodes, salivary glands, neck

[a] American Academy of Orofacial Pain classification.

that pain is a multidimensional experience encompassing sensory-discriminative, cognitive, motivational, and affective qualities. Suffering goes hand-in-hand with pain and is defined as the negative emotional and psychological state that occurs in response to or anticipation of nociception.[16] It is vital that the clinician remember that pain can be a symptom of the disease to be diagnosed and treated but may also be present in the absence of any physical findings. In essence, physical, psychological, and social factors are mutually influential forces that are able to create an infinite number of pain experiences for the patient.[17] A biologic system that includes anatomic, structural, and molecular substrates of disease interacts with a psychological and social system that includes the effects of motivation and personality on illness and an individual's reaction to it along with a cultural, environmental, and family influence on the expression and experience of pain.[18] Orofacial pain can be acute or chronic. Acute pain begins suddenly and usually does not last long, whereas chronic pain may last for weeks or months. Chronic pain is defined as pain that lasts for more than a month longer than expected based on the illness or injury. It may recur off and on for months and years and may be associated with a chronic disorder, such as cancer, diabetes, or fibromyalgia.[19]

Pain can also be divided into somatic and neuropathic pain. Somatic pain always results from stimulation of nociceptors, because of tissue injury, such as inflammation. Somatic pain ends, however, when underlying tissue injury and inflammation is resolved. The two hallmarks of somatic pain include hyperalgesia and allodynia.[20,21] Hyperalgesia is defined as an increased perception of the painful stimulus after receptor sensitization. Allodynia is the perception of pain in response to a nonnoxious stimuli. Neuropathic pain is considered pain that is initiated or caused by primary lesion or dysfunction in the nervous system.[22–25] Many of the kinds of orofacial pain discussed in this issue fall under this category. Treatment of them requires an understanding of neurophysiology of pain and the identification of sensible treatment goals. Specifically, treatment directed toward rehabilitation and pain control often supersedes treatment directed at a cure. Occasionally, pain may be of a psychogenic origin. Psychogenic pain is often unconscious, involuntary, and may accompany psychiatric disorders or may be an individual's way of dealing with the stresses of their mental illness.[26,27] It is an experience of mental suffering where there is no organic disease or where the organic disease has become overelaborated in its psychological, emotional, and behavioral significance.[27,28]

NEUROPHYSIOLOGY AND ANATOMY OF OROFACIAL PAIN

Nociceptors are responsible for the recognition of proprioception, mechanical stimuli, thermal stimuli, and pain perception.[29] Once stimulated, peripheral nerves direct nociceptive information and convey pain messages to the central nervous system by way of afferent fibers. Speed of transmission depends on the myelination and size of the nerve fibers. The three types of afferents include A, B, and C fibers. A fibers are myelinated and divided into alpha, beta, gamma, and delta. The A-delta fibers carry noxious stimuli that can damage tissues, such as the pain associated with heat. They are rapid conducting small fibers and are responsible for the initial pain of nociception. Fifty percent of C fibers carry afferent noxious stimuli and are polymodal. C fiber stimulation results in initial painless periods followed by diffuse and aching pains. In addition, C fiber nociception interconnects with the limbic system and plays a role in the emotional presentation of pain. In neuropathic pain chronic pain syndromes, the C fiber sensitizes a second high threshold neuron referred to as the wide dynamic range neuron leading to a condition often referred to as spinal windup.[30] This constant and continuous stimulation leads to facilitation of nonnoxious stimuli to a hyperalgesia state leading to relentless pain.[30] Pain can also be modulated by two primary types of drugs that work in the brain: analgesics and anesthetics.[31] The modulation of pain by electrical brain stimulation results from the activation of descending inhibitory fibers that modulate the input and output of various neurons.[30–32] In the central nervous system, much of the information from the nociceptive afferent fibers results from excitatory discharges of multireceptive neurons. The pain information in the central nervous system is controlled by ascending and descending inhibitory systems using endogenous opioids or other endogenous substances, such as serotonin, as inhibitory mediators.[33] In addition, a powerful inhibition of pain-related information occurs at the level of the spinal cord. These inhibitory systems can be activated by various mechanisms including brain stimulation, intracerebral morphine, and peripheral nerve stimulation. Many of the medications used in orofacial pain activate these inhibitory control mechanisms.[34]

To understand and effectively treat orofacial pain, the clinician must have a sound knowledge of the neuroanatomy and physiology of orofacial structures. Most nociceptive impulses are transmitted by the somatic nerves, a significant portion is transmitted by autonomic nerves, and a small portion may be transmitted by motor nerves. There are unique features of the oral and maxillofacial structures including the temporomandibular joint and masticatory muscles that make an understanding of the anatomy vital

---

Factors in pain modulation

- Nociceptors
  - Neuroeffector functions
  - Transmission of afferent signals
- Release of neurochemicals when nociceptors respond to noxious stimuli
  - Neuropeptides: substance P and CGRP
  - Excitatory AA: glutamate and aspartate
- Norepinephrine, bradykinin, serotonin, histamine, and prostaglandins
- Endogenous opioids work at receptors in the dorsal horn of the spinal cord and other areas
  - Three receptors: mu (m), kappa, and sigma
    - Most opioids bind to mu receptors
      - Subtype m1: analgesia
      - Subtype m2: respiratory depression, bradycardia, inhibition of gastrointestinal motility
    - Kappa: spinal analgesia without respiratory depression
    - Sigma: produces excitation and dysphoria
- Descending control
  - Responsible for arousal, attention, and emotional stress
  - Altering response to pain
- Modulation of dorsal horn
  - γ-Aminobutryic acid is thought to exert descending control by mediating presynaptic inhibition
  - Responsible for altering response to pain

in leading to appropriate diagnostic evaluation and management of patients with orofacial pain.[35,36]

The primary sensory innervation of the orofacial structures is the trigeminal system. The trigeminal system oversees the efficacy and tissue integrity of highly integrative orofacial behaviors that are controlled by the cranial nerves and modulated by the autonomic nervous system and greater limbic system.[32] Cranial nerves are extensions of the brain that innervate tissues involved with the trigeminal system directly or indirectly. The largest of the cranial nerves is the trigeminal nerve, which consists of three peripheral branches: (1) the ophthalmic, (2) the maxillary, and (3) the mandibular. Trigeminal nerve is the dominant nerve that relays sensory impulses from the orofacial area to the central nervous system. The regions where these branches collect sensory input conveyed by first-order neurons through the trigeminal ganglia encompass the entire face. The trigeminal nerve principally innervates facial skin, corneas, oral and nasal mucosa, teeth, tongue, masticatory muscles, and meningeal linings (**Fig. 1**). The trigeminal nerve has sensory and motor components. The sensory input converges into the spinal track nucleus of the brainstem.[31–34]

The facial nerve, glossopharyngeal nerve, and vagus nerves, and the upper cervical nerves 2 and 3 also relay sensory information from the face and surrounding area. The facial nerve has a large motor component that supplies the muscles of facial expression, platysma, stapedius, and scalp muscles in addition to a small sensory component that provides taste from the anterior tongue and parotid sensation. The glossopharyngeal nerve provides sensory efferent supply to the mucous membranes of the pharynx, palatine tonsils, and posterior tongue. The tympanic branch supplies sensory information from the middle ear, motor supply the muscles of the pharynx and soft palate, and special visceral afferents supply tastebuds of the posterior tongue. The upper for the five cervical nerves provide innervation to the back of the head,

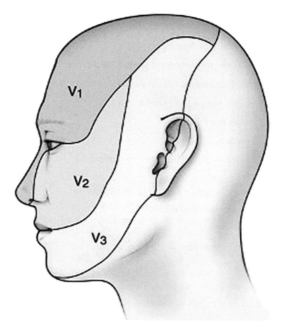

Fig. 1. Braches and innervation of the trigeminal nerve. (*From* Waldman S. Pain review. Philadelphia: Saunders Elsevier; 2009. p. 16; with permission.)

lower face, and neck. More importantly, they converge in the brainstem at the trigeminal nucleus (**Table 3**).

A common phenomenon associated with orofacial pain that often confuses the patient and the clinician is heterotopic pain.[37] One of the most important steps the clinician can take in the patient that presents with orofacial pain is determining the site of their pain and whether it coincides with the source of their pain. Primary pain occurs at the source and is often the case in acute injury or infection. This is not a difficult problem to diagnose and treat when other pain sources are absent. Diagnostic dilemmas are encountered and often unnecessary treatment performed when the source of pain is not located in the region of pain perception.[38] This phenomenon is referred to as heterotopic pain. The location where the patient feels the pain, which is easily located by asking the patient to point out the region of the body that is painful, is the site of pain. The source of the pain, however, is the area of the body from which the pain actually originates and may not necessarily be where the patient is experiencing pain. Another diagnostic challenge is referred pain. Referred pain describes pain felt at a location served by one nerve but the source of nociception arrives at the subnucleus caudalis by a different nerve. Convergence by multiple sensory nerves carrying input to the trigeminal spinal nuclei from cutaneous and deep tissues located throughout the head and neck sets the stage for referred pain. This convergence explains how intracranial, neck, shoulder, or throat nociception may actually excite second-order neurons receiving input from facial structures.[39]

Clinicians who evaluate and manage patients with orofacial pain realize a changing role as science clarifies how the central nervous system processes evolve when patients are exposed to chronic stressors. It is vital that practitioners get the entire story, which includes biomedical and psychosocial aspects of their patients' pain experience.[40]

Orofacial pain disorders comprise major and expensive components of health care in the United States. Collectively, they have a high prevalence rate and a large range in pain intensity with commensurate and often significant impact on the quality of life.[41] Ongoing basic and clinical research focused on acute and chronic orofacial pain

Table 3
Cranial and cervical nerves that provide somatic and visceral sensation to the orofacial area

Nerve	General Area Served
V: Trigeminal	Skin of the face, forehead, and scalp as far as the top of the head; conjunctiva and bulb of the eye; oral and nasal mucosa; part of the external aspect of the tympanic membrane; teeth; anterior two-thirds of the tongue; masticatory muscles; temporomandibular joint; meninges of the anterior and middle cranial fossae
VII: Facial	Skin of the hollow of the auricle of the external ear; small area of skin behind the ear
IX: Glossopharyngeal	Mucosa of the pharynx; fauces; palatine tonsils; posterior one-third of the tongue; internal surface of the tympanic membrane; skin of the external ear
X: Vagus	Skin at the back of the ear; posterior wall and floor of external auditory meatus; tympanic membrane; meninges of posterior cranial fossa; pharynx; larynx
Cervical nerve 2	Back of the head extending to the vertex; behind and above the ear; submandibular, anterior neck
Cervical nerve 3	Lateral and posterior neck

conditions is necessary to understand the unique features of this pain system and to develop and evaluate improved ways to treat patients with orofacial pain. Additional research is necessary to establish comprehensive classification schemes for all patients with orofacial pain.[42] It is encouraging to see current research studies incorporating quality-of-life indices, which provide important information on clinical outcomes for patients. The orofacial pain conditions reviewed in this issue represent a highly prevalent spectrum of pain disorders with pain intensities that are observed in many other pain conditions. It is clear, however, that there are unique anatomic, biochemical, and psychological components that provide compelling evidence for specific research and dedicated patient care on orofacial pain.

REFERENCES

1. Hargreaves KM. Orofacial pain. Pain 2011;152:S25–32.
2. Robert C, Wilson CS, Donnadieu S, et al. Bibliometric analysis of the scientific literature on pain research: a 2006 study. Pain 2008;138(2):250–4.
3. Robert C, Wilson CS, Donnadieu S, et al. Evolution of the scientific literature on pain from 1976 to 2007. Pain Med 2010;11(5):670–84.
4. Dworkin SF, LeResche L. Research diagnostic criteria for temporomandibular disorders: review, criteria, examinations and specifications, critique. J Craniomandib Disord 1992;6:301–55.
5. Benoliel R, Birman N, Eliav E, et al. The international classification of headache disorders: accurate diagnosis of orofacial pain? Cephalalgia 2008;28:752–62.
6. Anderson GC, Gonzalez YM, Ohrbach R, et al. The research diagnostic criteria for temporomandibular disorders. VI: future directions. J Orofac Pain 2010;24: 79–88.
7. Sternbach RA. Pain and 'hassles' in the United States: findings of the Nuprin pain report. Pain 1986;27(1):69–80.
8. Crook J, Tunks E, Rideout E, et al. Epidemiologic comparison of persistent pain sufferers in a specialty pain clinic and in the community. Arch Phys Med Rehabil 1986;67(7):451–5.
9. James FR, Large RG, Bushnell JA, et al. Epidemiology of pain in New Zealand. Pain 1991;44(3):279 83.
10. Lipton JA, Ship JA, Larach-Robinson D. Estimated prevalence and distribution of reported orofacial pain in the United States. J Am Dent Assoc 1993;124(10): 115–21.
11. Von Korff M, Dworkin SF, Le Resche L, et al. An epidemiologic comparison of pain complaints. Pain 1988;32(2):173–83.
12. Türp JC, Kowalski CJ, Stohler CS. Temporomandibular disorders–pain outside the head and face is rarely acknowledged in the chief complaint. J Prosthet Dent 1997;78(6):592–5.
13. Clauw DJ. Fibromyalgia: an overview. Am J Med 2009;122:S3–13.
14. Anastassaki A, Magnusson T. Patients referred to a specialist clinic because of suspected temporomandibular disorders: a survey of 3194 patients in respect of diagnoses, treatments, and treatment outcome. Acta Odontol Scand 2004;62:183–92.
15. Stohler CS. Chronic orofacial pain: is the puzzle unraveling? J Dent Educ 2001; 65(12):1383–92.
16. Hirshberg RM. Pain and suffering: a legal and medical lexicon for the 21st century. Med Law 2012;31(3):339–53.
17. Tenenbaum HC, Mock D, Gordon AS, et al. Sensory and affective components of orofacial pain: is it all in your brain? Crit Rev Oral Biol Med 2001;12(6):455–68.

18. Merrill RL. Central mechanisms of orofacial pain. Dent Clin North Am 2007;51(1): 45–59.
19. Arnold LM, Clauw DJ, Dunegan LJ, et al, FibroCollaborative. A framework for fibromyalgia management for primary care providers. Mayo Clin Proc 2012; 87(5):488–96.
20. Garland EL. Pain processing in the human nervous system: a selective review of nociceptive and biobehavioral pathways. Prim Care 2012;39(3):561–71.
21. Sessle BJ. Peripheral and central mechanisms of orofacial inflammatory pain. Int Rev Neurobiol 2011;97:179–206.
22. Iwata K, Imamura Y, Honda K, et al. Physiological mechanisms of neuropathic pain: the orofacial region. Int Rev Neurobiol 2011;97:227–50.
23. Baron R, Binder A, Wasner G. Neuropathic pain: diagnosis, pathophysiological mechanisms, and treatment. Lancet Neurol 2010;9(8):807–19.
24. Nickel FT, Seifert F, Lanz S, et al. Mechanisms of neuropathic pain. Eur Neuropsychopharmacol 2012;22(2):81–91.
25. Fornasari D. Pain mechanisms in patients with chronic pain. Clin Drug Investig 2012;32(Suppl 1):45–52.
26. Renton T, Durham J, Aggarwal VR. The classification and differential diagnosis of orofacial pain. Expert Rev Neurother 2012;12(5):569–76.
27. Aggarwal VR, Lovell K, Peters S, et al. Psychosocial interventions for the management of chronic orofacial pain. Cochrane Database Syst Rev 2011;(11):CD008456.
28. Williams AC, Eccleston C, Morley S. Psychological therapies for the management of chronic pain (excluding headache) in adults. Cochrane Database Syst Rev 2012;(11):CD007407.
29. Sacerdote P, Levrini L. Peripheral mechanisms of dental pain: the role of substance P. Mediators Inflamm 2012;2012:951920.
30. Staud R, Robinson ME, Price DD. Temporal summation of second pain and its maintenance are useful for characterizing widespread central sensitization of fibromyalgia patients. J Pain 2007;8(11):893–901.
31. Staud R. Abnormal endogenous pain modulation is a shared characteristic of many chronic pain conditions. Expert Rev Neurother 2012;12(5):577–85.
32. Ter Horst GJ, Copray J, Leim R, et al. Projections from the rostral parvocellular reticular formation to pontine and medullary nuclei in the rat: involvement in autonomic regulation and orofacial motor control. Neuroscience 1991;40:735–58.
33. Spetea M. Opioid receptors and their ligands in the musculoskeletal system and relevance for pain control. Curr Pharm Des 2013. [Epub ahead of print].
34. Bialer M. Why are antiepileptic drugs used for nonepileptic conditions? Epilepsia 2012;53(Suppl 7):26–33.
35. Benoliel R, Svensson P, Heir GM, et al. Persistent orofacial muscle pain. Oral Dis 2011;17(Suppl 1):23–41.
36. Bender SD. Temporomandibular disorders, facial pain, and headaches. Headache 2012;52(Suppl 1):22–5.
37. López-López J, Garcia-Vicente L, Jané-Salas E, et al. Orofacial pain of cardiac origin: review literature and clinical cases. Med Oral Patol Oral Cir Bucal 2012; 17(4):e538–44.
38. de C Williams AC, Cella M. Medically unexplained symptoms and pain: misunderstanding and myth. Curr Opin Support Palliat Care 2012;6(2):201–6.
39. Marfurt CF, Rajchert DM. Trigeminal primary afferent projections to "non-trigeminal" areas of the rat central nervous system. J Comp Neurol 1991;303(3):489–511.
40. Giamberardino MA, Affaitati G, Fabrizio A, et al. Myofascial pain syndromes and their evaluation. Best Pract Res Clin Rheumatol 2011;25(2):185–98.

41. Brattberg G, Parker MG, Thorslund M. A longitudinal study of pain: reported pain from middle age to old age. Clin J Pain 1997;13(2):144–9.
42. Mitchell LA, MacDonald RA. Qualitative research on pain. Curr Opin Support Palliat Care 2009;3(2):131–5.

Clinical Assessment of Patients with Orofacial Pain and Temporomandibular Disorders

Ilanit Stern, DMD[a],*, Martin S. Greenberg, DDS, FDS RCS[b]

KEYWORDS

- Orofacial pain • Temporomandibular disorder • Pain assessment
- Visual Analog Scale (VAS) • Numerical Rating Scale (NRS)
- Verbal Rating Scale (VRS) • McGill Pain Questionnaire (MPQ) • Diagnostic tests

KEY POINTS

- Accurate diagnosis of chronic pain disorders of the mouth, jaws, and face is frequently complex because there are multiple structures localized in 1 small anatomic region that can be a source of painful sensations. Pain can originate from multiple structures including teeth, sinus, eye, nerves, blood vessels, temporomandibular joint, and masticatory muscle sources.
- It is common for patients with chronic orofacial pain to consult multiple clinicians and receive an incorrect diagnosis and receive ineffective treatment before a correct diagnosis is reached. This problem is a significant public health concern when a serious or life-threatening disease is overlooked or a patient has chronic pain when effective therapy is available for the undiagnosed painful condition.
- Improved education in accurate diagnosis of orofacial disorders would not only decrease the number of patients with chronic pain but decrease the expense of unnecessary diagnostic tests and incorrect therapy.
- A clinician treating a patient with chronic orofacial pain can minimize error by starting the diagnostic procedure with the well-established method of a careful, accurate history and thorough head and neck examination followed by a thoughtfully constructed differential diagnosis.
- A careful, knowledgeable clinician minimizes incorrect diagnoses, unnecessary laboratory studies, and ineffective therapy. The possibility that the patient has symptoms or signs of a life-threatening underlying disease rather than the more common dental, sinus, or temporomandibular disorder must always be considered.

The authors have nothing to disclose.
a Department of Oral Health and Diagnostic Sciences, Center for Oral Medicine, College of Dental Medicine, Georgia Regents University, 1120 15th Street, Augusta, GA 30912, USA;
b University of Pennsylvania, School of Dental Medicine, 240 South 40th Street, Philadelphia, PA 19104, USA
* Corresponding author.
E-mail address: istern@gru.edu

Accurate diagnosis of chronic pain disorders of the mouth, jaws, and face is frequently complex because there are multiple structures localized in one small anatomic region that can be a source of painful sensations. Pain can originate from multiple structures including teeth, sinuses, eyes, nerves, blood vessels, temporomandibular joint (TMJ), and masticatory muscles.[1]

It is common for patients with chronic orofacial pain to consult multiple clinicians and receive an incorrect diagnosis and ineffective treatment before a correct diagnosis is reached. This problem is a significant public health concern when a serious or life–threatening disease is overlooked or a patient has chronic pain when effective therapy is available for their undiagnosed painful condition. Improved education in accurate diagnosis of orofacial disorders would not only decrease the number of patients with chronic pain but decrease the expense of unnecessary diagnostic tests and incorrect therapy.

A clinician treating a patient with chronic orofacial pain can minimize error by starting the diagnostic procedure with the well-established method of a careful, accurate history and thorough head and neck examination followed by a thoughtfully constructed differential diagnosis.[2] To reach a diagnosis, laboratory tests including imaging studies should be ordered only after a differential diagnosis containing likely causes of pain has been established based on the findings of the history and examination.

A careful, knowledgeable clinician will minimize incorrect diagnosis, unnecessary laboratory studies and ineffective therapy. The possibility that the patient has symptoms or signs of a serious life threatening underlying disease rather than the more common, dental, sinus or temporomandibular disorder must always be considered.

HISTORY

A complete history including past medical history, review of systems, family, and social history is essential, because each portion may lead to important information in a specific patient. A detailed history of the present illness is of particular importance in the diagnosis of the patient with chronic facial pain. The clinician should obtain a detailed story of the pain starting with the onset of symptoms including frequency, duration, quality (ie, burning, aching, lancinating), location, and severity.[3] Associated symptoms that may accompany the facial pain, as well as aggravating and alleviating factors, can provide valuable diagnostic information. It is helpful to ask the patient to rate the severity of the pain by the Visual Analog Scale (VAS). The past medical history should include items shown in **Table 1**.

The review of systems should be complete, with particular emphasis on symptoms of neurologic and musculoskeletal diseases. Symptoms such as facial numbness and weakness, paresthesia, diplopia, blurred vision suggesting a disease of the central nervous system (CNS) such as a brain tumor, aneurysm, or multiple sclerosis must be ruled out. Generalized muscle pain can be caused by fibromyalgia,[4,5] or pains in multiple joints suggests the possibility of rheumatoid arthritis or connective tissue disease in younger patients[6,7] or degenerative joint disease in the middle aged or elderly.[8]

Because psychological factors play an important role in several orofacial pain disorders, the review of systems as well as the family and social history is important to detect whether factors such as depression, anxiety, or increased stress at home or work may play a significant factor in chronic pain.[9]

PHYSICAL EXAMINATION

The physical examination includes a neurologic screening; general inspection of ears, nose, and oropharynx; TMJ; palpation of masticatory and cervical muscles; cervical

Table 1 Comprehensive history	
Chief complaint	Described in patients words
History of present illness	Chronology of onset Location of symptoms as pointed by patient Quality of symptoms: aching, dull, pressure pain most often represents musculoskeletal category, whereas throbbing, stabbing, pounding pain is neurovascular and burning, itching, electric shock–like pain describes neuropathic pain (some degree of overlap may occur) Timing, frequency, and duration (constant vs intermittent) Pain intensity can be measured by verbal rating (mild/moderate/sever), numeric rating (0–10), or VAS (10-cm line starting at 0 = no pain and ends at 10 = pain as bad as could be) Modifying factors that aggravate or alleviate pain (eg, chewing, light touch, emotional stress) Associated symptoms (eg, tearing; nasal congestion; nausea; vomiting; sensitivity to light, sounds, or motions; paresthesia; otalgia; headache)
Medical and dental history	Comorbid systemic disorders (eg, musculoskeletal, rheumatologic, and arthritic conditions) History of trauma to head and neck Parafunctional history: clenching, grinding History of previous treatments, and outcomes. Obtain information about medication dosage and length of treatment to avoid retreatment and determine whether previous treatment given was for the appropriate time and dose
Psychological and social history	Stressors and response to stress (social and occupational) Depression and anxiety are often comorbid factors Litigation, disability, and second gain Activity level and expectations

spine evaluation (posture and range of motion); and a detailed intraoral evaluation (summarized in **Table 2**).[10]

Musculoskeletal Evaluation

Musculoskeletal pain, primarily of the masticatory muscles, is the most prevalent cause of chronic pain of the orofacial region and is often overlooked by clinicians who do not include palpation of masticatory and neck muscles as part of the routine dental evaluation. Examination of these muscles for tenderness to palpation and pain referral may direct the clinician to the source of pain. Bilateral palpation of the masseters, deep and superficial temporalis, medial pterygoid, suprahyoid, mylohyoid, and anterior belly of the digastric muscles should be included in the examination. Palpation of the lateral pterygoid is unreliable because anatomically, it is nearly impossible to palpate.[11–13] Palpation may also reveal trigger points, which are hyperirritable sites in muscle taut bands. Provocation of trigger points causes significant discomfort and may refer pain to an adjacent location.[14,15]

Referred pain from the cervical muscles to the orofacial region is common[1] and palpation of cervical muscles should be included in a comprehensive assessment of orofacial pain.

Measurement of mandibular range of motion should include maximum comfortable opening, maximum unassisted opening regardless of pain, and assisted opening by gentle stretching. The range of lateral and protrusive movements should also be recorded. Cervical motion can be examined during active, passive, and resisted motions.

Table 2
Physical examination

System	Physical Examination	Examples of Related Disease
General appraisal	Asymmetry, swelling, tremors, posture Palpation of extraoral soft tissues such as lymph nodes and salivary glands	Neoplastic disease Dyskinesia Cervical spine disorders Multiple sclerosis
Musculoskeletal evaluation	Palpation of cervical and muscles of mastication. Palpation (and auscultation) of the TMJs for joint noises and their time of occurrence, tenderness, and swelling Measuring mandibular range of vertical and lateral movements. Inspect for corrected and uncorrected deviations, maximum opening with comfort, with pain, and passive range of motion (assisted opening) and signs of parafunction	Primary or secondary myalgia Myofacial pain Chronic widespread pain Localized arthritis Rheumatoid osteoarthritis Polyjoint osteoarthritis Disc displacement with or without reduction
Neurologic evaluation	Cranial nerve screening	CNS neoplasia Multiple sclerosis Secondary trigeminal neuralgia Chronic daily headaches Acute trigeminal neuritis
Vascular evaluation	Compression of temporal and carotid arteries	Temporal arteritis Trigeminal neuralgia caused by vascular compression
Ear, nose, and throat	Ear discharge, external lesions, swelling of parotid, external auditory canal examination by trained clinician, palpation of the maxillary and frontal sinuses, and visualization of oropharynx	Sinusitis Acute otitis media Neoplastic disease Parotid disease
Intraoral evaluation	Dental and periodontal examination Soft tissue condition (ulceration, mass, and infection) Stability of maxillomandibular relationship, and signs of parafunction	Vesiculobullous and ulcerative disease Dental disorders Periodontal disease

Palpation of the TMJs bilaterally in the closed position and during opening and closing movements can detect tenderness, pain, and joint sounds. Joint sounds can be associated with pain and limitation of mandibular range of motion indicating articular disk displacement, or arthritis. Joint sounds that are not associated with pain and dysfunction may be of little clinical significance and can be caused by functional adaptation of the disk to the TMJ.

In patients with unilateral throbbing headache, palpation for a tender, nodular temporal artery should be performed. If temporal arteritis is suspected, a complete blood count, erythrocyte sedimentation rate, and C-reactive protein should be ordered and referral for temporal artery biopsy may be indicated. Loss of vision in patients with undiagnosed temporal arteritis can be prevented with early use of systemic corticosteroids.[16]

Neurologic Examination

Screening of the cranial nerves should be part of the examination of a patient with orofacial pain to rule out a CNS lesion such as a tumor, aneurysm, or multiple sclerosis (cranial nerve motor and sensory functions are listed in **Table 3**). Specific detailed examination of the sensory and motor functions of the trigeminal nerve is essential for a patient with chronic pain. A positive finding of motor or sensory dysfunction along a distribution of a cranial nerve necessitates additional investigation such as magnetic resonance imaging (MRI) of the brain and consultation with a neurologist or neurosurgeon.

Ear, Nose, and Throat

Pain caused by sinusitis or other abnormalities of the paranasal sinuses, such as tumors, can be referred to different parts of the head. Maxillary sinusitis can project to the malar, palate, and teeth.[17] Palpation of the maxillary sinuses for tenderness, percussion of the maxillary posterior teeth for general tenderness, Valsalva maneuver, and bending forward are helpful diagnostic methods of detecting pain from sinusitis.

It is common for patients who have a TMD to present with otalgia or tinnitus, and they are often referred by an otolaryngologist after a normal examination to rule out dental disease or TMD.

Intraoral Evaluation

Intraoral examination includes inspection of the soft tissue for lesions, ulcerations, swellings, and masses. Additional testing such as pulp testing, percussion, and testing for tooth mobility may follow when an intraoral examination for a suspected odontogenic

Table 3
Cranial nerve function

Cranial Nerve	Function
I. Olfactory	Sense of smell
II. Optic	Visual acuity, visual fields
III. Oculomotor	Movement of eyeball, pupil, and upper eyelid
IV. Trochlear	Eye movement
V. Trigeminal	Tactile facial sensation, motor innervation of muscle of mastication, corneal reflex
VI. Abducens	Lateral movements of the eyes
VII. Facial	Movement of facial muscles Extrinsic and intrinsic ear muscles, taste (anterior two-thirds of tongue)
VIII. Acoustic vestibular	Hearing, equilibrium and orientation of head in space
IX. Glossopharyngeal	Elevation of palate, movement of pharynx and larynx. General sensation from palate, posterior one-third of tongue, and oropharynx. Taste from posterior one-third of tongue and oropharynx
X. Vagus	Muscles of soft palate, base of tongue, pharynx, larynx. Parasympathetic fibers to thoracic and abdominal viscera
XI. Accessory	Movement of sternocleidomastoid and trapezius muscles
XII. Hypoglossal	Movement of the tongue

source of pain is required. When indicated, dental occlusion should be evaluated for wear facets, although this may be an unreliable assessment of parafunction.[16]

Pain arising from salivary glands is usually well localized, can be more pronounced during eating, and is accompanied by swelling of the gland. The salivary glands should be palpated and tenderness noted. Milking the salivary glands for production of normal clear saliva from the major salivary gland ducts should also be included in the routine examination.

PAIN ASSESSMENT METHODS

Measurement of pain assists the clinician in the process of differential diagnosis and of evaluation of treatment effectiveness. The pain experience is subjective and, as such, cannot be objectively measured by a single test. Most of the assessment methods for orofacial pain rely on the patient's ability to express the experience of pain via questionnaire, diary, or interview. The verbal communication of pain poses a challenge because different individuals may describe and rate the intensity of pain of similar biomedical quality in different manners. No correlation was found in chronic pain conditions between tissue injury and related degree of pain.[18] Pain is not only an unpleasant sensory experience but also involves a subjective emotional response. As such, it can be expressed in different ways. Verbal communication of pain complaint, facial and body expression, social dysfunction, and physical dysfunction may all be displayed in one individual, whereas another individual may complain less but use facial expression, and a third person may exhibit social or physical dysfunction. Pain is therefore considered to be a multidimensional entity in which the impact of pain on a patient's life and degree of disability are important to consider when planning treatment.

SELF-RATING INSTRUMENTS FOR MEASUREMENT OF PAIN
Pain Intensity Measurement

Pain intensity measurements are used to quantify patients' estimated severity of pain. Visual analogue scale (VAS), Numerical Rating Scale (NRS), and Verbal Rating Scale (VRS) are the most common methods of rating pain intensity.

A VAS is a linear scale on which patients specify their level of pain by indicating the position along a continuous 10-cm line between 2 end points: 0 cm indicates no pain and 10 cm indicates that the pain is as bad as it could be. The distance from the low end of the VAS to the patient's mark is measured as a numerical index of the severity of pain. VAS can also be used to measure the effect of pain. The patient is asked to rate the unpleasantness of the pain experience: 0 cm indicates not bad at all, and 10 cm indicates the worst unpleasant feeling imaginable. The validity and sensitivity of VAS is well established.[19] For potential greater sensitivity, VAS could be drawn on a 10-cm line having 101 response levels (0–100). A disadvantage of VAS is the requirement of the patient to have a minimal level of motor skill and visual and cognitive ability, in particular in abstract thought. VAS is more difficult to understand than other measures of pain intensity, especially among individuals at risk for cognitive difficulties,[20,21] such as elderly individuals and patients on high doses of opioids. Herr and colleagues[22] argued that failure to use the VAS correctly was related to educational level, cognitive impairment, and motor abilities, and not age, per se. Using an NRS involves asking the patient to rate the pain from 0 to 10 or from 0 to 100, with the understanding that 0 represents no pain and 10 or 100 represents pain as bad as it could be. The patient chooses the number that best corresponds with the intensity of pain. NRS has good sensitivity, is easy to administer, and generates data that can be statistically analyzed.[23] It is particularly useful with geriatric patients and patients with impaired motor skills. The primary weakness of NRS is that it may not have ratio qualities.[24]

Ratio quality is the direct correlation between the magnitude of the pain and the line length or the numerical representation. Although this may not affect the reliability of the treatment outcome, the clinician cannot conclude that a change from 7 to 6 in NRS represents 10% decrease in perceived pain. The scale that has ratio quality is VAS.[25]

A VRS consists of a series of verbal pain descriptions from least to most intense. Many different VRS lists have been created with adjectives that describe gradual change in pain intensity. For example, in a 4-point scale used by Seymore,[26] no pain is given a score of 0; mild pain, 1; moderate, 2; and severe pain a score of 3. This method is simple for patients to understand, and is the preferred pain scale for older adults because it requires that patients interpret and express their pain in verbal terms.[27] However, VRS can be time consuming when patients need to review a long list of adjectives before rating their pain if using a 15-point scale. VRS is less reliable among illiterate patients. It also lacks ratio quality. The interval between 0 (no pain) and 1 (mild pain) can be different from that between 1 (mild pain) and 2 (moderate pain).[19] All rating scales can be used at the time of initial assessment and during treatment to track treatment outcomes.

Assessing Pain Experience

The McGill Pain Questionnaire (MPQ) is a widely used self-rating instrument for measurement of pain in clinical and research settings. The MPQ, which is based on the gate control theory,[28] was designed to provide a multidimensional assessment of pain that takes into consideration the motivational-affective and cognitive-psychological aspects along with the sensory physiologic aspects.[29]

The questionnaire contains 16 groups of adjectives describing increasing degrees of sensory, affective, and evaluative qualities. An additional 4 groups are dedicated to the location and temporal characteristics of pain and the rating of present pain intensity. The MPQ was shown to be valuable as an aid to diagnosis. It can emphasize the difference between pain syndromes. For instance assessment by the MPQ finds the quality of pain of burning mouth syndrome different from toothache pain, whereas the magnitude is equal.[30] In addition, MPQ was shown to be valuable as a single overall measure of pain magnitude when studying pain mechanisms and efficacy of pain interventions.[31,32]

Assessing Adjustment to Pain

A patient and a clinician can view the success of treatment differently. For the patient, reduction of pain may be the primary goal of the treatment, whereas, for a clinician, success of treatment may be defined as pain reduction and restoration of function. In some patients with chronic pain, reduction of pain is difficult to achieve and restoring function becomes the main criterion for judging treatment success.

Dworkin and LeResche[33] recognized the impact of factors such as jaw disability, psychological status, and psychosocial functioning in assessment of patients with TMD. They proposed the research diagnostic criteria (RDC) for evaluation of patients with TMD that focuses on 2 axes, for the purpose of TMD clinical research. Axis I comprises the clinical examination and diagnostic classification of TMD. Axis II includes the assessment of patients' TMD pain–related behavioral functioning, psychological status, and adaptation to pain. Dworkin and LeResche used the Graded Chronic Pain Severity (GCPS) scale to assess psychosocial function, the Depression Scale and Vegetative Symptom Scale from the Symptom Checklist-90-Revised (SCL-90-R) for assessment of psychological status, and a jaw disability checklist.[34,35] All the scales listed earlier are based on questionnaires that are completed by the patient. The GCPS scale assesses chronic pain severity from grade 0 to grade IV, and is designed to capture the extent to which the pain is disabling. It is a useful clinical measure to assess the impact of TMD on patients in population-based studies. The questionnaire comprises 7 questions, of which 3 are related to pain intensity and 4 are related to disability. The SCL-90-R depression scale is used to identify patients with chronic pain who may be experiencing significant depression, anxiety, and somatization. These conditions are common among patients with chronic orofacial pain, and represent risk factors for long-term persistence of TMD pain.[36] Moreover, preexisting psychosocial characteristics represent risk factors for new-onset TMD.[37]

Not all orofacial patients require a comprehensive psychological assessment such as SCL-90-R, Minnesota Multiphasic Personality Inventory, or West Haven–Yale Multidimensional Pain Inventory as part of the examination. However, the clinician needs to be aware of certain conditions that possibly initiate or maintain chronic orofacial pain, and screen for depression, anxiety, stressful life events, secondary gain, and overuse of the health system (**Box 1**). Patients who require a more comprehensive psychological assessment should be referred for an evaluation by a psychiatrist or psychologist.

DIAGNOSTIC TESTS
Diagnostic Imaging

All diagnostic tests are not routinely indicated for every patient. Use of a specific test depends on the differential diagnosis after the history and examination have been completed and evaluated.[38] In other instances, imaging is used to screen for unsuspected pathology or to recognize disease stage or assess treatment effectiveness.[39,40] To choose the most appropriate test for the patient, the clinician needs to consider the cost, potential benefits, radiation dose, and availability of various imaging techniques. First the clinician must decide what type of information is needed to aid in the diagnosis and management of the patient. MRI is most specific and sensitive for interpretation of soft tissue and inflammatory conditions in the joint,[41,42] whereas plain films, panoramic radiographs, conventional and computed tomography portray the osseous morphology and disorders of the joint with variable degrees of detail.[41] The expected findings in each modality and the effect on treatment should dictate the most appropriate modality to be chosen in a given situation (diagnostic imaging for TMD and orofacial pain is discussed elsewhere in this issue). As mentioned earlier,

---

Box 1
Considerations when screening for behavioral and psychological factors during pain assessment

- Disability in daily work, household maintenance, and recreational and social activities that is out of proportion to objective findings
- Symptoms of psychological disorders: depression, anxiety, somatization
- Prolonged or excessive use of opiates, benzodiazepines, alcohol, or other drugs
- Evidence of secondary gain
- Major life events and variation of pain depending on those events
- Repeated failure to conventional therapy
- Symptoms incompatible with innervation pathway
- Other chronic pain elsewhere in the body

MRI is an effective imaging modality in the diagnosis of disc position and configuration, disc perforation, joint effusion, osseous and bone marrow changes in the TMJ,[41,42] but no publication has reported diagnostic thinking efficacy or therapeutic efficacy.[43]

Imaging is a critical diagnostic tool when a tumor is suspected. Because orofacial pain can be a manifestation of benign or malignant tumors,[44–46] it is common to use imaging to rule out CNS, salivary gland, and bony and soft tissue masses, by respective diagnostic modality. For instance, brain MRI could be helpful in ruling out CNS disorders when there is:

- Pain associated with sensory loss in the region of the trigeminal nerve
- Repetitive abnormal movement of jaw, lips, tongue
- Involuntary contractions, paralysis, or weakness of facial or jaw muscles
- Sudden onset of severe headache in an adult
- Facial pain accompanied by diplopia, loss of vision, or dysphagia

Because approximately 10% of patients with symptoms of trigeminal neuralgia have underlying CNS disorders, MRI of the brain with thin sections through the brain is indicated when the patient presents with the typical electriclike lancinating pain.

LABORATORY TESTING

Laboratory tests are only indicated when certain conditions are suspected. **Table 4** lists these conditions. Most orofacial pain and TMD disorders do not cause abnormalities that can be identified in the laboratory, and most laboratory tests are used to rule out an underlying disease such as a neoplasm, cranial arteritis, or systemic disease.

Table 4 Laboratory testing	
Suspected Disease	**Laboratory Testing**
Temporal arteritis	ESR Temporal artery biopsy
Rheumatoid arthritis	Complete blood cell count RF CCP ANA ESR CRP test
Systemic lupus erythematous	Complete blood cell count ANA Anti-dsDNA antibody Anti-Sm antibody RF Anti-SSA Anti-SSB Urinalysis ESR CRP test Serum complements Biopsy

Abbreviations: ANA, antinuclear antibody; CCP, cyclic citrullinated peptide antibody; CRP, C-reactive protein; ESR, erythrocyte sedimentation rate; RF, rheumatoid factor.

DIAGNOSTIC NERVE BLOCK

A diagnostic nerve block can be helpful in establishing a diagnosis, particularly when used to distinguish peripheral disease, such as a dental disorder, from more centrally acting neuropathic pain. If pain does not resolve after a nerve block, then the neuropathic changes are likely to be central in origin.[47] The clinician should use the information gathered from diagnostic nerve blocks with caution for several reasons[48,49]:

- Local anesthetics may induce systemic effects
- Proximity of other neural structures to the nerve, ganglion, or plexus being blocked may lead to the inadvertent and often unrecognized block of adjacent nerves, invalidating the results that the clinician sees
- Placebo effects
- Technical limitations that limit the ability to perform an accurate diagnostic nerve block
- Anatomic variations that may influence the results
- Patients fearing the procedural pain may premedicate themselves before diagnostic nerve blocks

A diagnostic nerve block can be hard to interpret and should always be considered in the context of all of the clinical findings.[49]

REFERENCES

1. Bereiter DA, Hargreaves KM, Hu JW. Trigeminal mechanisms of nociception: peripheral and brainstem organization. In: Bushnell MC, editor. The senses, a comprehensive reference. San Diego (CA): Academic Press; 2008. p. 435–60.
2. Lund JP, Widmer CG, Feine JS. Validity of diagnostic and monitoring tests used for temporomandibular disorders. J Dent Res 1995;74(4):1133–43.
3. Okeson JP. Bell's orofacial pains. The Clinical Management of Orofacial Pain. Chicago: Quintessence; 2005.
4. Fraga BP, Santos EB, Farias Neto JP, et al. Signs and symptoms of temporomandibular dysfunction in fibromyalgic patients. J Craniofac Surg 2012;23(2):615–8.
5. Yunus MB. The prevalence of fibromyalgia in other chronic pain conditions. Pain Res Treat 2012;2012:584573.
6. Klasser GD, Balasubramaniam R, Epstein J. Topical review-connective tissue diseases: orofacial manifestations including pain. J Orofac Pain 2007;21(3): 171–84.
7. Aliko A, Ciancaglini R, Alushi A, et al. Temporomandibular joint involvement in rheumatoid arthritis, systemic lupus erythematosus and systemic sclerosis. Int J Oral Maxillofac Surg 2011;40(7):704–9.
8. Alexiou K, Stamatakis H, Tsiklakis K. Evaluation of the severity of temporomandibular joint osteoarthritic changes related to age using cone beam computed tomography. Dentomaxillofac Radiol 2009;38(3):141–7.
9. Dworkin SF. Behavioral characteristics of chronic temporomandibular disorders: diagnosis and assessment. In: Sessle BJ, Bryant PS, Dionne RA, editors. Temporomandibular disorders and related conditions. Seattle (WA): IASP Press; 1995. p. 175–92.
10. Clark GT, Seligman DA, Solberg WK, et al. Guidelines for the examination and diagnosis of temporomandibular disorders. J Craniomandib Disord 1989;3(1):7–14.
11. Johnstone D, McCormick J. The feasibility of palpating the lateral pterygoid muscle. J Prosthet Dent 1980;44:318.

12. Conti PC, Dos Santos Silva R, Rossetti LM, et al. Palpation of the lateral pterygoid area in the myofascial pain diagnosis. Oral Surg Oral Med Oral Pathol Oral Radiol Endod 2008;105(3):e61–6.
13. Stratmann U, Mokrys K, Meyer U, et al. Clinical anatomy and palpability of the inferior lateral pterygoid muscle. J Prosthet Dent 2000;83(5):548–54.
14. Hong CZ, Kuan TS, Chen JT, et al. Referred pain elicited by palpation and by needling of myofascial trigger points: a comparison. Arch Phys Med Rehabil 1997;78(9):957–60.
15. Wright EF. Manual of temporomandibular disorders. Ames (IA): Blackwell; 2005.
16. Blasberg B, Eliav E, Greenberg MS. Orofacial pain. In: Greenberg MS, Glick M, Ship JA, editors. Burket's oral medicine, vol. 10, 11th edition. Hamilton Ontario: BC Decker; 2008. p. 257–88.
17. Silberstein SD. Headaches due to nasal and paranasal sinus disease. Neurol Clin 2004;22:1–19.
18. Turk D, Rudy T. Toward a comprehensive assessment of chronic pain patients. Behav Res Ther 1987;25:237–49.
19. Jensen MP, Karoly P. Self reported scales and procedures for assessing pain in adults. In: Turk DC, Melzack R, editors. Handbook of pain assessment. vol. 2. New York: Guilford Press; 2011. p. 19–44.
20. Jensen MP, Karoly P, Braver S. The measurement of clinical pain intensity: a comparison of six methods. Pain 1986;27(1):117–26.
21. Paice JA, Cohen FL. Validity of a verbally administered numeric rating scale to measure cancer pain intensity. Cancer Nurs 1997;20(2):88–93.
22. Herr K, Spratt K, Mobily P, et al. Pain intensity assessment in older adults: use of experimental pain to compare psychometric properties and usability of selected pain scales with younger adults. Clin J Pain 2004;20(4):207–19.
23. Williamson A, Hoggart B. Pain: a review of three commonly used pain rating scales. J Clin Nurs 2005;14(7):798–804.
24. Price DD, Bush FM, Long S, et al. A comparison of pain measurement characteristics of mechanical visual analogue and simple numerical rating scales. Pain 1994;56(2):217–26.
25. Price DD, McGrath PA, Rafii A, et al. The validation of visual analogue scales as ratio scale measures for chronic and experimental pain. Pain 1983;17(1):45–56.
26. Seymour RA. The use of pain scales in assessing the efficacy of analgesics in post-operative dental pain. Eur J Clin Pharmacol 1982;23(5):441–4.
27. Herr K, Mobily P. Comparison of selected pain assessment tools for use with the elderly. Appl Nurs Res 1993;6:39.
28. Melzack R, Wall P. Pain mechanisms: a new theory. Science 1965;150:971–9.
29. Melzack R. The McGill Pain Questionnaire: major properties and scoring methods. Pain 1975;1:277–99.
30. Grushka M, Sessle BJ, Miller R. Pain and personality profiles in burning mouth syndrome. Pain 1987;28:155–67.
31. Reading AE. Testing pain mechanisms in persons in pain. In: Wall PD, Melzack R, editors. Textbook of pain. Edinburgh (United Kingdom): Churchill Livingstone; 1984. p. 195–204.
32. Sharav Y, Singer E, Schmidt E, et al. The analgesic effect of amitriptyline on chronic facial pain. Pain 1987;31:199–209.
33. Dworkin SF, LeResche L. Research diagnostic criteria for temporomandibular disorders: review, criteria, examinations and specifications, critique. J Craniomandib Disord 1992;6:302–55.

34. Von Korff M, Ormel J, Keefe FJ, et al. Grading the severity of chronic pain. Pain 1992;50:133–49.
35. Derogatis L. SCL-90-R: administration, scoring and procedures manual - II for the revised version. Towson (MD): Clinical Psychometric Research; 1983.
36. Garofalo JP, Gatchel RJ, Wesley AL, et al. Predicting chronicity in acute temporomandibular joint disorders using the research diagnostic criteria. J Am Dent Assoc 1998;129:438–47.
37. Fillingim R, Ohrbach R, Greenspan J, et al. Potential psychosocial risk factors for chronic TMD: descriptive data and empirically identified domains from the OPPERA Case-Control Study. J Pain 2011;12(Suppl 11):T46–60.
38. Lindvall AM, Helkimo E, Hollender L, et al. Radiographic examination of the temporomandibular joint. A comparison between radiographic findings and gross and microscopic morphologic observations. Dentomaxillofac Radiol 1976;5(1–2):24–32.
39. Hatcher DC. Craniofacial imaging. J Calif Dent Assoc 1991;19(6):27–34.
40. Eliasson S, Isacsson G. Radiographic signs of temporomandibular disorders to predict outcome of treatment. J Craniomandib Disord 1992;6(4):281–7.
41. Brooks SL, Brand JW, Gibbs SJ, et al. Imaging of the temporomandibular joints, position paper of the American Academy of Oral and Maxillofacial Radiology. Oral Surg Oral Med Oral Pathol Oral Radiol Endod 1997;93:609–18.
42. Larheim TA, Westesson PL, Sano T. MR grading of temporomandibular joint fluid: association with disk displacement categories, condyle marrow abnormalities and pain. Int J Oral Maxillofac Surg 2001;30:104–12.
43. Ribeiro-Rotta RF, Marques KD, Pacheco MJ, et al. Do computed tomography and magnetic resonance imaging add to temporomandibular joint disorder treatment? A systematic review of diagnostic efficacy. J Oral Rehabil 2011;38(2): 120–35.
44. Dodick D. Headache as a symptom of ominous disease. Postgrad Med 1997; 101:46 62.
45. Stodulski D, Mikaszewski B, Stankiewicz C. Signs and symptoms of parotid gland carcinoma and their prognostic value. Int J Oral Maxillofac Surg 2012;41(7): 801–6.
46. Clark GT, Ram S. Orofacial pain and neurosensory disorders and dysfunction in cancer patients. Dent Clin North Am 2008;52(1):183–202.
47. Merrill RL. Orofacial pain mechanisms and their clinical application. Dent Clin North Am 1997;41:167–88.
48. Sethna N, Berde C. Diagnostic nerve blocks: caveats and pit-falls in interpretation. IASP News 1995;3–5.
49. Steven D. Waldman. Guide to Pain Management in Low-Resource Settings: Diagnostic and Prognostic Nerve Blocks. IASP 2010. Available at: http://www.iasp-pain.org/AM/Template.cfm?Section=Home&Template=/CM/ContentDisplay.cfm&ContentID=12172.

Diagnostic Imaging for Temporomandibular Disorders and Orofacial Pain

Allison Hunter, DMD, MS[a],*, Sajitha Kalathingal, BDS, MS[b]

KEYWORDS

- Imaging • Cone beam computed tomography • CBCT • Orofacial pain
- Temporomandibular disorders • Diagnostic imaging • Temporomandibular joint

KEY POINTS

- Research diagnostic criteria for temporomandibular disorders (RDC/TMD) were established and published in 1992. The RDC/TMD recommend arthrography and magnetic resonance imaging (MRI) for disk displacement and tomography for evaluation of bony changes. Since the establishment of the RDC/TMD, additional imaging techniques have become available. In addition, a section specifically designed to describe image analysis is lacking in both the original and the updated RDC/TMD.

- Diagnostic imaging, when indicated, is an important part of the examination process for TMD and orofacial pain patients. Imaging may be used to confirm suspected disease, rule-out disease, and gather additional information when the clinical diagnosis is equivocal or unclear. Certain historical and clinical presentations increase the likelihood of positive findings on imaging examinations. Examples of such findings include the presence of a reciprocal click, a closed lock, and crepitus.

- The ability to assess details in multiplanar views makes cone beam computed tomography a unique tool for accurate and precise evaluation of dento-alveolar structures. The spatial resolution has tremendously improved with the new generation cone beam computed tomography scanners in which flat panel detectors are used in place of image intensifiers and charged couple devices.

- Advanced imaging with computed tomography or MRI may be indicated for orofacial pain patients presenting with idiopathic facial pain, headaches, or trigeminal neuralgia. The suspected cause of clinical symptoms would influence the imaging examination ordered. It has been suggested that MRI be routinely ordered for trigeminal neuralgia patients to rule out potential causes of secondary (symptomatic) trigeminal neuralgia.

The authors have nothing to disclose.
[a] Department of Oral Health and Diagnostic Sciences, College of Dental Medicine, Georgia Regents University, GC 2248, 1120 15th Street, Augusta, GA 30912-1241, USA; [b] Department of Oral Health and Diagnostic Sciences, College of Dental Medicine, Georgia Regents University, GC 2252, 1120 15th Street, Augusta, GA 30912-1241, USA
* Corresponding author.
E-mail address: ahunter@gru.edu

INTRODUCTION
Nature of the Problem

As many as 50% of elderly people may be affected by orofacial pain.[1] Due to the complexity of the nature of the pain and diverse etiology, it is often hard to diagnose and treat this condition.

Definition

Orofacial pain may be attributed to a variety of disorders including atypical idiopathic facial pain, temporomandibular disorders (TMD), diseases of odontogenic or soft tissue origin, neuralgia, and headaches. TMD is considered to be the main cause of pain in the orofacial region following pain of odontogenic origin. Diseases affecting the temporomandibular joint (TMJ) can be divided as articular disease and disease affecting the ligaments and musculature of the joint. Articular disease affecting the hard tissue includes the osseous and cartilaginous structures as well as the joint space. Congenital and developmental disorders, neoplasia, internal derangements of the articular disk, inflammatory diseases, systemic diseases, ankylosis, and fracture all are pathoses included under articular diseases. Myalgia related to the TMJ is often linked to parafunctional habits and psychosocial and behavioral changes.

Diagnostic Dilemmas

Research diagnostic criteria for temporomandibular disorders (RDC/TMD) were established and published in 1992.[2] The RDC/TMD details the clinical and historical assessment of TMD patients in an effort to standardize these processes for improved reliability and validity of TMD research. The RDC/TMD recommend arthrography and magnetic resonance imaging (MRI) for disk displacement and tomography for evaluation of bony changes. Since the establishment of the RDC/TMD, additional imaging techniques have become available. In addition, a section specifically designed to describe image analysis is lacking in both the original and the updated RDC/TMD.[3]

The focus of this article is diagnostic imaging used for evaluation of TMD and orofacial pain. For additional information on cranial neuralgias and the clinical evaluation of the orofacial pain patient, the respective articles on these topics should be referred to.

Rationale for Imaging

Diagnostic imaging, when indicated, is an important part of the examination process for TMD and orofacial pain patients. Imaging may be used to confirm suspected disease, rule-out disease, and gather additional information when the clinical diagnosis is equivocal or unclear. Certain historical and clinical presentations increase the likelihood of positive findings on imaging examinations. Examples of such findings include the presence of a reciprocal click, a closed lock, and crepitus.[2] Indications for diagnostic imaging are summarized in **Box 1**.

Imaging Modalities

1. Two-dimensional
   - Conventional tomography
   - Transcranial, transmaxillary, transpharyngeal projections
   - Submentovertex projection
   - Posteroanterior and lateral cephalometric projections
   - Panoramic radiography
     - Open and closed views

2. Three-dimensional
   - Multislice computed tomography (MSCT)
   - Cone beam computed tomography (CBCT)
   - Magnetic resonance imaging (MRI)

Box 1
Indications for diagnostic imaging of the TMJ
Trauma
Changes in occlusion
Limitation of opening/closed lock
Presence of reciprocal click
Crepitus
Systemic diseases
Swelling/infection
Failure of conservative treatment

Table 1 provides a list of advantages and disadvantages of these imaging modalities.

Table 1
Advantages and disadvantages of different imaging modalities used to evaluate the TMJ

Imaging Modality	Advantages	Disadvantages
Conventional tomography	Optional technique on panoramic units, accessibility	Does not depict subtle osseous changes or soft tissues, technique sensitive
Transcranial, transmaxillary, transpharyngeal projections	These techniques were used in the past to evaluate gross osseous changes	Do not depict subtle osseous changes or soft tissues, technique sensitive, limited trained personnel
Submentovertex projection	Optional technique on panoramic units	Provides limited diagnostic information
Posteroanterior and lateral cephalometric projections	Low radiation dose	Provides limited diagnostic information for TMJ
Panoramic radiography including open and closed views of the TMJ	Availability, expense, low radiation dose	Does not depict subtle osseous changes or soft tissues
Multislice computed tomography (MSCT)	Availability, 3-dimensional technique	High radiation dose
Cone beam computed tomography (CBCT)	Typically low radiation dose relative to MSCT, 3-dimensional technique	Availability, variable radiation dose based on imaging parameters, advanced training for interpretation
Magnetic resonance imaging (MRI)	Depicts soft tissue and osseous changes, uses nonionizing radiation, 3-dimensional technique	Time, expense, certain metallic implants preclude use, pacemakers preclude use

IMAGING MODALITIES FOR HARD TISSUE EVALUATION
Panoramic Radiography

The original RDC/TMD and updated RDC/TMD do not list panoramic radiography as an imaging option for evaluation of the TMD patient.[2–4] Perhaps this is because panoramic radiography depicts only the lateral poles and central parts of the condyle and is only useful when there are marked changes in osseous structures.[4–6] Ahmad and colleagues[4] demonstrated the poor sensitivity of panoramic radiographs in which only 26% displayed imaging findings of osteoarthritis when compared with computed tomography (CT). However, when orofacial pain is thought to arise from an odontogenic cause, panoramic imaging may be very useful.[5] **Fig. 1** gives an example of the utility of panoramic imaging. Panoramic units may also be equipped with a TMJ imaging program. This TMJ program allows image acquisition at a more appropriate angle through the condyle in open and closed views. The x-ray beam is angled through the long axis of the condyle and the image layer thickness is decreased in the TMJ imaging mode (refer to **Fig. 2**).

CBCT

CBCT was introduced to dentistry in 1998.[7] The machine design is similar to a panoramic unit with the detector and the x-ray source located 180° apart. The scanning is performed by rotating the x-ray source and detector synchronously around the head of the patient. The patient may be seated, standing, or supine and must remain still until the image acquisition is complete. Several hundreds of sequential planar projection images (2-dimensional basis images) are acquired during this rotation and the data are reconstructed by the computer using specific algorithms. The image acquisition time may vary from 5 to 40 seconds; however, due to a technology named pulsed mode exposure, radiation is not always emitted continuously, but only during a fraction of the total imaging time, significantly reducing the radiation dose to the patient and one of the main advantages of CBCT over medical CT.

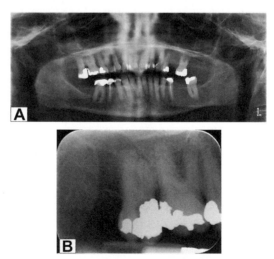

Fig. 1. Odontogenic source of orofacial pain. (*A*) Panoramic image depicts overhangs on teeth nos. 2 and 3. In addition, the peri-apical region of the mesiobuccal root of no. 2 appears abnormal. (*B*) Peri-apical image of the area reveals suspected recurrent decay and a peri-apical radiolucency on the mesiobuccal root of no. 2.

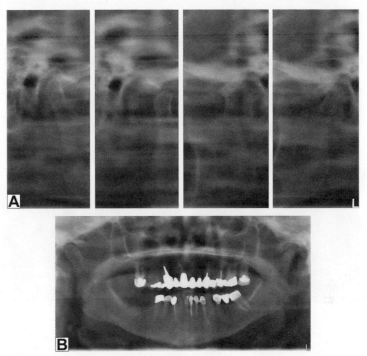

Fig. 2. Panoramic TMJ imaging program. (*A*) TMJ imaging program open and closed views. (*B*) Standard panoramic image of the same patient for comparison.

Watanabe and colleagues[8] found that small-volume CBCT produced high-quality images at a fraction of the radiation dose of MSCT. It has been estimated that CBCT exposures are 10% or less of medical CT.[9] CBCT examinations may also be lower in dose than conventional 2-dimensional imaging commonly used in dentistry. In some cases a TMJ examination acquired with CBCT can be accomplished at one-half the effective dose of an intra-oral full-mouth series radiographic examination.[10,11] It should be noted however that the dose of CBCT is variable. The dose associated with CBCT varies according to many factors, such as the size of the field of view, the area of the maxillofacial complex imaged, the spatial resolution selected, the number of basis projections acquired, and the use of continuous versus pulse-beam exposure. When considering the more commonly used CBCT manufacturers, radiation dose may vary from approximately 4 to 10 panoramic radiographs.[10–13]

The ability to assess details in multiplanar views makes CBCT a unique tool for accurate and precise evaluation of dento-alveolar structures. The spatial resolution has tremendously improved with the new generation CBCT scanners in which flat panel detectors are used in place of image intensifiers and charged couple devices. Spatial resolution is isotropic and ranges from 0.076 to 0.4 mm. The high spatial resolution of CBCT allows for the evaluation of early bony changes in the TMJ.[14,15] CBCT has also been shown to perform better than conventional tomography, panoramic radiography, and MSCT for the evaluation of the components of the TMJ.[4,14,16] **Fig. 3** provides a comparison of panoramic radiography and CBCT of the TMJ. **Fig. 4** demonstrates TMJ imaging with conventional panoramic radiography, panoramic TMJ open and closed views, and CBCT.

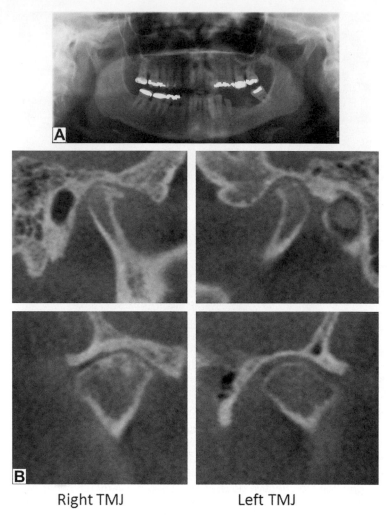

Right TMJ   Left TMJ

Fig. 3. Evaluation of the TMJ with panoramic radiography and CBCT. (*A*) Panoramic radiograph demonstrates flattening of the condyle and the posterior slope of the articular eminence on the right side. (*B*) CBCT depicts osteophyte formation and subchondral erosion of the right condyle, which are not appreciated in the panoramic image.

IMAGE ANALYSIS—HARD TISSUE
Osseous Tissue

When evaluating the hard tissues of the TMJ, it is important to assess the overall shape of the condyle and fossa and to confirm that the cortical borders are uniform and intact. Due to adaptive remodeling or disease process affecting the joint, the hard tissue changes on the images may be depicted as flattening, sclerosis, osteophyte formation, erosion, and presence/absence of loose bodies within the joint space.

Osteoarthritis (Degenerative Joint Disease)

Along with internal derangement, osteoarthritis (OA) is one of the most common diseases of the TMJ.[17,18] The incidence of OA increases with age and demonstrates a

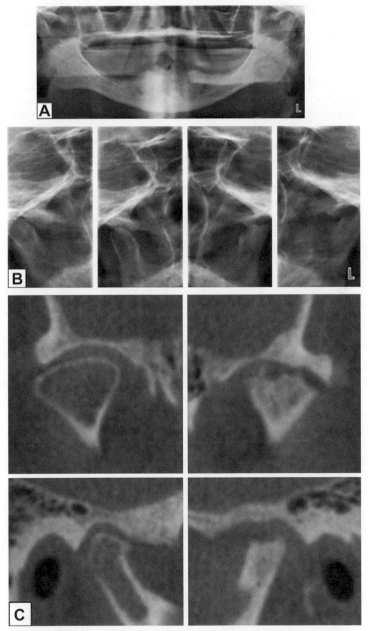

Fig. 4. Evaluation of gross morphologic changes of the left condyle and fossa with conventional panoramic radiography, panoramic TMJ views, and CBCT. (*A*) Panoramic radiograph. (*B*) Panoramic TMJ open and closed views. (*C*) CBCT corrected coronal and sagittal views.

female predilection.[17,19,20] Although acute trauma, hypermobility, and parafunction have been suggested as possible causes, only 10% of the population experiences pain.[17,20] Osseous proliferative changes, such as osteophyte formation and generalized sclerosis, and osseous degenerative changes, such as erosion and subchondral cyst formation, are indicative of OA.[17,19,20] The incidence of osseous changes is higher in the presence of long-term nonreducing disks.[17,20] Minimal flattening of the condyle and/or eminence and localized sclerosis should be regarded as remodeling and should not be confused with OA.[4,5,21]

Inflammatory Joint Disease

Rheumatoid arthritis (RA) is a systemic autoimmune disease usually presenting with bilateral and symmetric polyarticular involvement.[20,22,23] This disease involves pannus formation, which constitutes a proliferative reaction of the synovium.[22,23] RA is more common in women and typically occurs in the fourth and fifth decades of life.[20,22,23] Symmetric involvement of the hands and feet is common and occurs before changes in the TMJ.[20,23,24] Disease-related changes in the TMJ may range from severe erosion to complete destruction of the condylar head and even ankylosis.[20,24,25] **Fig. 5** demonstrates the severe condylar resorption that can occur with RA. **Fig. 6** demonstrates the difference in imaging findings associated with OA and RA. In addition to RA, ankylosing spondylitis and psoriatic arthropathy are systemic arthritides also defined by inflammation of the synovial membrane.[20,21] Ankylosing spondylitis and psoriatic arthropathy rarely affect the TMJ and imaging findings are similar to those of RA.[20,21,24]

Joint Space Calcifications

Calcifications within the joint space can be seen with OA and RA.[20,24] However, it should be kept in mind that the cause of joint space calcifications may also include synovial chondromatosis, chondrocalcinosis, osteochondritis dissecans, and metastatic calcifications. Of these, synovial chondromatosis is one of the more common causes of calcifications of the joint space and many patients with synovial chondromatosis of the TMJ present with symptoms of TMD.[26,27]

Position of Condyle Within Glenoid Fossa

Posterior positioning of the condyles has been applied as a radiographic indicator of anterior disk displacement and has been found with higher frequency in symptomatic populations.[2,6] Rammelsberg and colleagues[28] found that subjects with bilateral anterior disk displacement with reduction demonstrated posterior condylar positioning. In a study population of TMD subjects of which 69% demonstrated anterior disk displacement with or without reduction, there was a preference for posterior positioning of the condyles.[29]

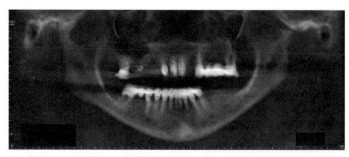

Fig. 5. Effects of rheumatoid arthritis (RA) on the condyle. Panoramic reconstruction using CBCT demonstrates that the left condyle has been completely resorbed by RA. (*Courtesy of Dr Kirk Young, DDS, MS, Orange Park, FL*).

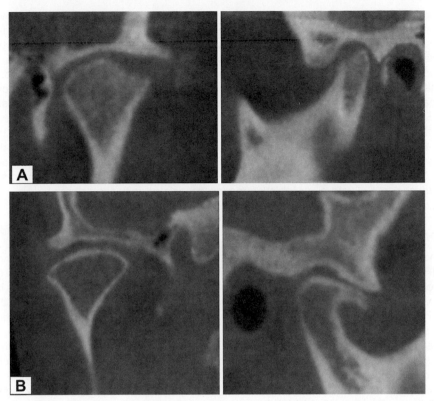

Fig. 6. Comparison of the effects of RA and osteoarthritis (OA) (also known as Degenerative Joint Disease) on the TMJ. (*A*) CBCT corrected coronal and sagittal views of a patient with RA. The CBCT findings on the left condyle demonstrate the characteristic erosive nature of RA. (*B*) CBCT corrected coronal and sagittal views of a patient with OA. The CBCT findings on the right condyle demonstrate the characteristic proliferative nature of OA.

Ren and colleagues[30] found that a posterior positioning of the condyle was favored in patients with anterior disk displacement, particularly in nonreducing joints; however, the positioning of the condyles in normal individuals was fairly evenly distributed between anterior, posterior, and centric positioning. In a systematic review by Stamm and colleagues,[31] it was shown that a comparison of publications with the highest level of evidence demonstrated no statistically significant difference in condylar position (centric vs anterior-superior vs posterior) in asymptomatic individuals; however, a trend for centric positioning was noted. In the American Academy of Oral and Maxillofacial Radiology position paper, it states that the clinical significance of condylar nonconcentricity is unclear because of the literature reporting a high variability in condylar position.[5] It is important to bear in mind when evaluating condylar concentricity on imaging that the condyle may be posterior or anterior in position in normal joints.[30] Therefore, although one may suspect anterior disk displacement when observing posterior condylar positioning on imaging, correlation with MRI and/or clinical findings is needed to confirm.

IMAGE ANALYSIS—MRI

Larheim[21] reported that disk displacement is found in approximately 80% of patients imaged for TMD, the most common being anterior disk displacement. MRI has superior soft tissue differentiation because of its improved contrast resolution over conventional tomography and CBCT.[32] Therefore, MRI is used to evaluate the soft tissue components of the TMJ. MRI may be used to evaluate the position of the disk, the shape of the disk, the signal of the disk, the presence/absence of fluid within the joint space (joint effusion), the marrow signal of the condyle, the presence of loose bodies within the joint, pannus formation (in the case of inflammatory arthritides), and osseous changes. An imaging protocol that may be used for MRI of the TMJ is proton density (PD) and T2-weighted sequences acquired in corrected sagittal and coronal views with use of TMJ surface coils.[4,18,21,33] Translation can be evaluated by imaging the maximum opening on the sagittal PD images; it is not necessary to acquire the open views on both sequences.[4] Another option is to use T1-weighted sequences in place of PD-weighted sequences.[17,29] Contrast may be used on T1-weighted sequences to evaluate synovial inflammation associated with the arthritides (eg, RA, psoriatic arthropathy, and ankylosing spondylitis).[5,21]

TMJ Evaluation with MRI

The articular disk demonstrates a biconcave morphology and a low signal intensity on MRI due to its fibrous tissue nature.[33] In the closed-mouth position, the disk should be located with its posterior band superior to the condyle (12 o'clock position) and its intermediate zone over the anterior prominence of the condyle.[21,33] However, the normal location of the posterior band of the disk may not always assume a 12 o'clock position and some have used the 11 o'clock position of the disk to define anterior displacement.[29] The bone marrow of the condyle should normally appear as a homogeneous high (bright) signal on T1-weighted or proton density–weighted sequences and as a homogeneous intermediate signal on T2-weighted sequences.[21,33,34] An example of normal and abnormal marrow signal is provided in **Fig. 7**. A low signal on T1-weighted or PD-weighted sequences and a high signal on T2-weighted sequences would suggest marrow edema.[34] A low signal on T1-weighted or PD-weighted sequences and T2-weighted sequences would suggest marrow sclerosis or fibrosis.[34] A heterogenous marrow signal may indicate osteonecrosis.[21,34] Although uncertain, disk displacement has been suggested as a possible cause of osteonecrosis.[26,34] A minimal amount of joint effusion may be regarded as normal.[18,34,35]

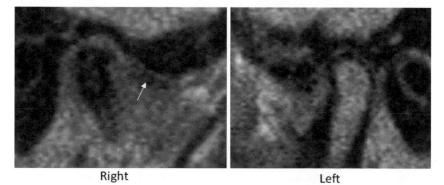

Right   Left

Fig. 7. PD-weighted closed-mouth corrected sagittal view of the right and left TMJ. The left condyle demonstrates the normal marrow signal observed on PD images, whereas the right condyle demonstrates low signal due to sclerosis. There is also flattening and osteophyte formation on the right condyle and anterior displacement of the disc (*arrow*) on the right side.

However, more than minimal joint effusion is seen often in conjunction with internal derangement (with or without reduction) and may often be accompanied by pain.[18]

IMAGING MODALITIES FOR EVALUATION OF OROFACIAL PAIN

Advanced imaging with CT or MRI may be indicated for orofacial pain patients presenting with idiopathic facial pain, headaches, or trigeminal neuralgia. The suspected cause of clinical symptoms would influence the imaging examination ordered. It has been suggested that MRI be routinely ordered for trigeminal neuralgia (TN) patients to rule out potential causes of secondary (symptomatic) TN.[36] Secondary TN may be due to compression of the trigeminal nerve by tumors, cysts, vascular anomalies, or due to multiple sclerosis.[36] The reported most common imaging finding in TN is vascular compression of the nerve root and is subsequently the most common cause for classical TN.[37–39] Evaluation for neurovascular compression with MRI has a reported high sensitivity and specificity.[40,41] Lacerda Leal and colleagues[40] reported that 3D T2 high-resolution, 3D time of flight magnetic resonance angiography (TOF-MRA), and 3D T1 with gadolinium (contrast-enhanced) sequences are the preferred MRI examinations for identifying a neurovascular compression. Diffusion-weighted MRI has also been used.[37,42] In addition to arteries, veins can serve as the source of compression for the trigeminal nerve root.[40,41] Lacerda Leal and colleagues[40] used a combination of 3D TOF-MRA and contrast-enhanced MRI sequences to differentiate the 2 vessel types.

Because the trigeminal nerve exits the pons in the cerebellopontine angle (CPA) cistern, tumors and cysts arising in this area may cause compression of the trigeminal nerve.[39] Schwannomas, meningiomas, and epidermoid cysts make up most (approximately 99%) of CPA cistern lesions.[43] Vestibular schwannomas account for most CPA tumors, contributing to 65% to 85% of all tumors.[43,44] MRI and CT may be used to evaluate these CPA cistern lesions. CT is especially useful for the evaluation of bony changes associated with meningiomas and schwannomas. Meningiomas may cause hyperostosis or erosion of the adjacent bone.[45] Vestibular schwannomas or meningiomas may cause widening of the porus acusticus of the internal auditory canal.[43,45] Calcifications are present in 25% of meningiomas, which can be appreciated on CT.[46] Thickening of the dura surrounding meningiomas may occur and is best evaluated with contrast-enhanced MRI.[44] MRI is preferred to CT for the evaluation of the cranial nerves in cases of vestibular schwannomas and in some cases is used to predict hearing loss after surgery.[44] The cystic nature of epidermoid cysts can be confirmed by observing lack of contrast enhancement on CT or MRI. In addition, multiple sclerosis and vascular aneurysms may cause symptoms of trigeminal neuralgia. In the case of multiple sclerosis, MRI is used for assessment of white matter lesions.[46,47] Conventional angiography, computed tomography angiography, and TOF-MRA may be used to assess vascular aneurysms.

Headaches (HA) are another indication for advanced imaging. A severe HA with sudden onset, a new-onset HA, a migraine of adult onset, cluster HA, and a change in nature of the HA[39,48] are all potential indications for brain imaging. HA may indicate the presence of tumors, aneurysms, or arteriovenous malformations.[48] Depending on the nature of the cause of HA, CT or MRI or both may be necessary for diagnosis.

REFERENCES

1. Shinal RM, Fillingim RB. Overview of orofacial pain: epidemiology and gender differences in orofacial pain. Dent Clin North Am 2007;51(1):1–18.

2. Dworkin SF, LeResche L. Research diagnostic criteria for temporomandibular disorders: review, criteria, examinations and specifications, critique. J Craniomandib Disord 1992;6:301–55.

3. Department of Oral Medicine Orofacial Pain Research Group. Research diagnostic criteria for temporomandibular disorders. Seattle (WA): University of Washington; 2011. p. 1–29.

4. Ahmad M, Hollender L, Anderson Q, et al. Research diagnostic criteria for temporomandibular disorders (RDC/TMD): development of image analysis criteria and examiner reliability for image analysis. Oral Surg Oral Med Oral Pathol Oral Radiol Endod 2009;107:844–60.

5. Brooks SL, Brand JW, Gibbs SJ, et al. Imaging of the temporomandibular joint: a position paper of the American Academy of Oral and Maxillofacial Radiology. Oral Surg Oral Med Oral Pathol Oral Radiol Endod 1997;83:609–18.

6. Petersson A. What you can and cannot see in TMJ imaging – an overview related to the RDC/TMD diagnostic system. J Oral Rehabil 2010;37:771–8.

7. Mozzo P, Procacci C, Tacconi A, et al. A new volumetric CT machine for dental imaging based on the cone-beam technique: preliminary results. Eur Radiol 1998;8:1558–64.

8. Watanabe H, Hondab E, Tetsumuraa A, et al. A comparative study for spatial resolution and subjective image characteristics of a multi-slice CT and a cone-beam CT for dental use. Eur J Radiol 2011;77:397 402.

9. Zinman EJ, White SC, Tetradis S. Legal considerations in the use of cone beam computer tomography imaging. J Calif Dent Assoc 2010;38(1):49–56.

10. Ludlow JB, Ivanovic M. Comparative dosimetry of dental CBCT devices and 64-slice CT for oral and maxillofacial radiology. Oral Surg Oral Med Oral Pathol Oral Radiol Endod 2008;106:106–14.

11. Ludlow JB, Davies-Ludlow LE, White SC. Patient risk related to common dental radiographic examinations: the impact of 2007 International Commission on radiological protection recommendations regarding dose calculation. J Am Dent Assoc 2008;139:1237–43.

12. Scarfe WC, Levin MD, Gane D, et al. Use of cone beam computed tomography in endodontics. Int J Dent 2009;1–20. http://dx.doi.org/10.1155/2009/634567.

13. Ludlow JB. A manufacturer's role in reducing the dose of cone beam computed tomography examinations: effect of beam filtration. Dentomaxillofac Radiol 2011; 40:115–22.

14. Bartling SH, Majdani O, Gupta R, et al. Large scan field, high spatial resolution flat-panel detector based volumetric CT of the whole human skull base and for maxillofacial imaging. Dentomaxillofac Radiol 2007;36:317–27.

15. Barghan S, Tetradis S, Mallya S. Application of cone beam computed tomography for assessment of the temporomandibular joints. Aust Dent J 2012; 57(Suppl 1):109–18.

16. Honey OB, Scarfe WC, Hilgers MJ, et al. Accuracy of cone-beam computed tomography imaging of the temporomandibular joint: comparisons with panoramic radiology and linear tomography. Am J Orthod Dentofacial Orthop 2007;132: 429–38.

17. De Leeuw R, Boering G, Van Der Kuijl B, et al. Hard and soft tissue imaging of the temporomandibular joint 30 years after diagnosis of osteoarthrosis and internal derangement. J Oral Maxillofac Surg 1996;54:1270–80.

18. Westesson PL, Brook SL. Temporomandibular joint: relationship between MR evidence of effusion and the presence of pain and presence of pain and disk displacement. AJR Am J Roentgenol 1992;159:559–63.

19. Wiberg B, Wanman A. Signs of osteoarthrosis of the temporomandibular joints in young patients: a clinical and radiographic study. Oral Surg Oral Med Oral Pathol Oral Radiol Endod 1998;86:158–64.
20. Petrikowski CG. Diagnostic imaging of the temporomandibular joint. In: White SC, Pharoah MJ, editors. Oral radiology. Principles and interpretation. 6th edition. St Louis (MO): The C.V. Mosby Company; 2008. p. 473–505.
21. Larheim TA. Role of magnetic resonance imaging in the clinical diagnosis of the temporomandibular joint. Cells Tissues Organs 2005;180:6–21.
22. Treister N, Glick M. Rheumatoid arthritis: a review and suggested dental care considerations. J Am Dent Assoc 1999;130:689–98.
23. Neville BW, Damm DD, Allen CM, et al. Oral and maxillofacial pathology. 3rd edition. St Louis (MO): Saunders Elsevier; 2009. p. 878–80.
24. Mafee MF, Valvassori GE, Becker M. Valvassori's imaging of the head and neck. Revised and enlarged. 2nd edition. New York: Thieme; 2005. p. 494–5.
25. Oynther GW, Tronje G, Holmlund AB. Radiographic changes in the temporomandibular joint in patients with generalized osteoarthritis and rheumatoid arthritis. Oral Surg Oral Med Oral Pathol Oral Radiol Endod 1996;81:613–8.
26. Campos PS, Freitas CE, Pena N, et al. Osteochondritis dissecans of the temporomandibular joint. Dentomaxillofac Radiol 2005;34:193–7.
27. Ida M, Yoshitake H, Okoch K, et al. An investigation of magnetic resonance imaging features in 14 patients with synovial chondromatosis of the temporomandibular joint. Dentomaxillofac Radiol 2008;37:213–9.
28. Rammelsberg R, Jäger L, Pho Duc JM. Magnetic resonance imaging-based joint space measurements in temporomandibular joints with disk displacements and in controls. Oral Surg Oral Med Oral Pathol Oral Radiol Endod 2000;90: 240–8.
29. de Senna BR, Marques LS, França JP, et al. Condyle-disk-fossa position and relationship to clinical signs and symptoms of temporomandibular disorders in women. Oral Surg Oral Med Oral Pathol Oral Radiol Endod 2009;108: e117–24.
30. Ren YF, Isberg A, Westesson PL. Comparison between asymptomatic volunteers with normal disk position and patients with disk displacement. Oral Surg Oral Med Oral Pathol Oral Radiol Endod 1995;80:101–7.
31. Stamm T, Hohoff A, Meegen AV, et al. On the three-dimensional physiological position of the temporomandibular joint. J Orofac Orthop 2004;65:280–9.
32. Curry TS, Dowdey JE, Murry RC. Christensen's physics of diagnostic radiology. 4th edition. Philadelphia: Lippincott Williams & Wilkins; 1990. p. 432–504.
33. Westesson PL, Yamamoto M, Seno T, et al. Temporomandibular joint. In: Som PM, Curtin HD, editors. Head and neck imaging. 4th edition. St Louis (MO): Mosby; 2003. p. 995–1054.
34. Larheim TA, Westesson PL, Hicks DG, et al. Osteonecrosis of the temporomandibular joint: correlation of magnetic resonance imaging and histology. J Oral Maxillofac Surg 1999;57:888–98.
35. Larheim TA, Westesson PL, Sano T. MR grading of temporomandibular joint fluid: association with disk displacement categories, condyle marrow abnormalities and pain. Int J Oral Maxillofac Surg 2001;30:104–12.
36. Goru SJ, Pemberton MN. Trigeminal neuralgia: the role of magnetic resonance imaging. Br J Oral Maxillofac Surg 2009;47:228–9.
37. Lutz J, Linn J, Mehrkens JH, et al. Trigeminal neuralgia due to neurovascular compression: high-spatial-resolution diffusion—tensor imaging reveals microstructural neural changes. Radiology 2011;258(2):524–30.

38. Yip V, Michael BD, Nahser HC, et al. Arteriovenous malformation: a rare cause of trigeminal neuralgia identified by magnetic resonance imaging with constructive interference in steady state sequences. QJM 2012;105:895–8.
39. Siccoli MM, Bassetti CL, Sándor PS. Facial pain: clinical differential diagnosis. Lancet Neurol 2006;5:257–67.
40. Lacerda Leal PR, Hermier M, Froment JC, et al. Preoperative demonstration of the neurovascular compression characteristics with special emphasis on the degree of compression, using high-resolution magnetic resonance imaging: a prospective study, with comparison to surgical findings, in 100 consecutive patients who underwent microvascular decompression for trigeminal neuralgia. Acta Neurochir 2010;152:817–25.
41. Lacerda Leal PR, Hermier M, Souza MA. Visualization of vascular compression of the trigeminal nerve with high-resolution 3T MRI: a prospective study comparing preoperative imaging analysis to surgical findings in 40 consecutive patients who underwent microvascular decompression for trigeminal neuralgia. Neurosurgery 2011;69:15–26.
42. Trebbastoni A, D'Antonio F, Biasiotta A, et al. Diffusion tensor imaging (DTI) study of a trigeminal neuralgia due to large venous angioma. Neurol Sci 2013;34(3): 397–9.
43. Bonneville F, Savatovsky J, Chiras J. Imaging of cerebellopontine angle lesions: an update. Part 1: enhancing extra-axial lesions. Eur Radiol 2007;17:2472–82.
44. Marcel Maya M, Lo WW, Kouvanlikaya I. Temporal bone: tumors and cerebellopontine angle lesions. In: Som PM, Curtin HD, editors. Head and neck imaging. 4th edition. St Louis (MO): Mosby; 2003. p. 1275–360.
45. Mafee MF, Valvassori GE, Becker M. Valvassori's Imaging of the Head and Neck. Second edition revised and enlarged. New York: Thieme; 2005. p. 97–8; 269–71.
46. Tintoré M, Rovira A, Martínez MJ, et al. Isolated demyelinating syndromes: comparison of different MR imaging criteria to predict conversion to clinically definite multiple sclerosis. AJNR Am J Neuroradiol 2000;21:702–6.
47. Barkhof F, Filippi M, Miller DH, et al. Comparison of MRI criteria at first presentation to predict conversion to clinically definite multiple sclerosis. Brain 1997;120: 2059–69.
48. Detsky ME, McDonald DR, Baerlocher MO, et al. Does this patient with headache have a migraine or need neuroimaging? JAMA 2006;296:1274–83.

Differential Diagnosis of Orofacial Pain and Temporomandibular Disorder

Anil Kumar, DMD*, Michael T. Brennan, DDS, MHS

KEYWORDS

- Differential diagnosis • Orofacial pain • TMD • Headache • Pain

KEY POINTS

- Orofacial pain can have a variety of sources.
- Always begin with a broad differential diagnosis.
- Rule out rare but serious causes before investigating minor causes.
- Be wary of omitting a condition from the differential diagnosis until sufficient information rules it out.

INTRODUCTION

In the dental community, complaints of pain in the head and neck region are certainly a common reason why patients seek treatment. Dental professionals need to be thorough when assessing a patient presenting with pain, including obtaining a detailed and comprehensive history of present illness, past medical history, social history, as well as performing a systematic, thorough clinical examination. After all of this information is collected, the next crucial step is creating a differential diagnosis.

Formulating a complete differential diagnosis involves creating a list of conditions that could be causing a patient's pain. For the new practitioner, this is time-consuming; however the benefit of being overly inclusive far outweighs the risk of missing or mistreating a diagnosis due to lack of critical thinking on the front end. In many instances, common conditions can be appropriately dealt with in a quick manner (eg, localized pain related to a clearly carious tooth), but there are more serious conditions that can mimic the nonspecific pain of less-threatening entities. These outliers should not be discounted.

Department of Oral Medicine, Carolinas Medical Center, PO Box 32861, Charlotte, NC 28232, USA
* Corresponding author.
E-mail address: anil.kumar@carolinas.org

Dent Clin N Am 57 (2013) 419–428
http://dx.doi.org/10.1016/j.cden.2013.04.003
0011-8532/13/$ – see front matter
dental.theclinics.com

Because many orofacial pain conditions can cause diffuse, non-specific, or referred pain, correlating the history with the clinical examination becomes a critical task. This ensures that all contributing factors and subjective signs are taken into consideration along with the objective findings. As the list of possible diagnoses is systematically reviewed, conditions should be omitted accordingly when ruled out. A provider should not remove a potential diagnosis until ample data support it being dismissed. Additionally, a differential diagnosis can change after initial triage. The list should be dynamic to keep up-to-date information and prevent oversight of conditions that were not originally included, but were subsequently incorporated with additional diagnostic information. Furthermore, duration can be an important factor in maintaining a potential diagnosis, as acute and chronic pain can lead the clinician in a different direction to determine the underlying etiology.

DIFFERENTIAL DIAGNOSIS

In this article, a brief outline of the various causes of orofacial pain is listed in addition to key information and classic signs and symptoms of each of these etiologies. The etiologies are broken down into the following categories[1]

- ○ Intracranial pain
- ○ Headaches
- ○ Neuropathic pain
- ○ Intraoral pain
- ○ Temporomandibular disorders
- ○ Cervical pain
- ○ Pain related to anatomically associated structures
- ○ Referred pain
- ○ Psychiatric and mental illness (psychogenic)

Many of these etiologies will be elaborated upon in other articles in this issue. Tables are included in some of the sections, listing the common characteristics of certain disorders. For other sections, tables are not included, since these are conditions that are less commonly managed by dental practitioners.

Intracranial Pain

Although the vast majority of patients who present to an outpatient dental clinic may not have pain related to an intracranial etiology, these entities should always be considered due to their level of severity and potential for serious adverse events.[1] Possible causes of intracranial pain include, but are not limited to

- ○ Tumors (benign or malignant)
- ○ Aneurysm
- ○ Intracranial bleeding (hemorrhage or hematoma)
- ○ Intracranial swelling or edema
- ○ Abscess or infection

If a provider believes that a patient's pain could possibly be caused by anything in the previous lists, the patient should be referred for further testing and immediate treatment, as these causes are potentially life threatening. Signs and symptoms that should lead one to be suspicious of an intracranial cause of pain include

- ○ Acute onset with rapidly progressing severity
- ○ Severe sleep disturbances
- ○ Exacerbation of pain due to positional changes

- Neurologic deficits (eg, speech difficulties, memory loss, forgetfulness, loss of cognition)
- New onset of seizures
- Vertigo
- Partial or complete paralysis
- Ataxia
- Constitutional symptoms (eg, fever, fatigue, weight loss, malaise, chills, night sweats)

Although some of these signs and symptoms could be caused by less serious or other underlying disease processes, including and/or ruling out intracranial causes should not be overlooked.

Headaches—Primary or Secondary

Even if a dental provider is not directly managing primary headache disorders, it is important to have a working knowledge of the common entities, including

- Migraine
- Cluster headache
- Tension-type headache
- Trigeminal autonomic cephalgias (TACs)
- Paroxysmal hemicrania
- Temporal arteritis

Migraine headaches are usually unilateral, pulsatile, and accompanied by photophobia and/or phonophobia. Additionally, patients may present with a prodromal aura. Cluster headaches are located primarily in the orbital and temporal region, with accompanying lacrimation, swelling of the forehead or eyelid, and possible rhinorrhea. Paroxysmal hemicrania presents similar to a cluster headache, except that it is shorter in duration. Tension-type headaches are neurovascular in etiology, more diffuse, with dull aching pain, and in general are bilateral. All of these conditions will be discussed in further detail in other articles in this issue. Headaches can also be secondary to any of the primary causes of orofacial pain discussed in this and other articles.

Given that many patients who present to dental professionals may have the previously mentioned conditions, it is important to have a working knowledge of them, and place them on the differential diagnosis if necessary. Some orofacial pain patients may present with headaches secondary to some of the other conditions covered in this article (eg, pain from a toothache causing a headache), and in this case the dental professional may be indirectly managing a patient's headache symptoms via treatment of the primary source (**Table 1**).

Neuropathic

Neuropathic pain arises from disturbances in the nervous system. These abnormalities can occur centrally, peripherally, or at both levels. They can be idiopathic or secondary to trauma or illness. Additionally, neuropathic pain can be episodic, continuous, or a combination of both. Two of the more common episodic neuropathic pain conditions include trigeminal neuralgia and glossopharyngeal neuralgia.

Of note, an episodic neuralgia can occur in other nerves of the orofacial region, and they are named according to the nerve that supplies sensory information to the affected area. These neuralgias usually present as paroxysmal sharp, shooting pain that lasts a short duration (seconds to minutes). The triggers can be unknown, but

Table 1
Differential diagnosis of headaches

Condition	Signs and Symptoms
Migraine[2,3]	• Prodromal symptoms—euphoria, depression, irritability, food cravings, constipation, neck stiffness, increased yawning • Aura—visual, sensory, verbal, and/or motor disturbances • Throbbing and pulsatile • Photophobia and phonophobia • Long duration
Cluster Headache (Subclassification of TAC)[4–6]	• Orbital and temporal regions • Short-lived • Unilateral • Autonomic symptoms—ptosis, miosis, lacrimation, rhinorrhea, nasal congestion
Tension-type[7]	• Diffuse, dull, aching pain • Bilateral • Precipitated by stress and mental tension
Paroxysmal Hemicrania (subclassification of TAC)[8]	• Unilateral • Shorter-lived than cluster headaches (lasts 2–30 minutes) • Most often in V1 distribution • Orbital, temporal, and frontal regions • Abrupt onset and cessation • Similar autonomic symptoms as cluster headaches
Temporal arteritis[9]	• Age >50 y • Localized headache of new onset • Tenderness or decreased pulse of the temporal artery • Erythrocyte sedimentation rate >50
Other TACs	• SUNCT (short-lasting unilateral neuralgiform headache attacks with conjuntival injection and tearing) • SUNA (short-lasting unilateral neuralgiform headache attacks with cranial autonomic symptoms)

pain can result from direct stimulation of the affected area. Common causes of continuous neuropathic pain include

- Postherpetic neuralgia
- Pain resulting from trauma (aberrant healing of nerve tissue or development of neuromas)
- Burning mouth syndrome
- Atypical odontalgia
- Atypical facial pain/persistent idiopathic facial pain

As opposed to classic neuralgias, continuous neuropathic pain frequently presents as burning that can be accompanied by paresthesia, dysesthesia, and/or allodynia. It may be difficult to determine clinically whether the etiology of this pain is central or peripheral if no distinct aggravating or precipitating factors can be elicited. If this is the case, then further radiographic evaluation, laboratory testing, or referral could be warranted (**Table 2**).

Intraoral

Pain related to the oral cavity is probably the most frequent complaint of patients seeking dental treatment.[1,20] Intraoral pain can be referred (eg, myofascial pain

Table 2 **Differential diagnosis of neuropathic pain**	
Condition	**Signs and Symptoms**
Trigeminal neuralgia[10,11]	• Paroxysmal, intense, sharp, and shooting pain • Short-lived pain (seconds) • Unilateral • V2 and V3 distributions commonly involved • Frequently has triggers such as chewing, talking, brushing teeth, cold air, smiling, or touching of trigger zones
Glossopharyngeal neuralgia[11]	• Paroxysmal, intense, sharp, and shooting pain • Short-lived pain (seconds) • Unilateral • Areas innervated by CN IX and CNX are affected—ear, tonsillar fossa, base of tongue, and the area beneath the angle of the mandible • Less common than trigeminal neuralgia • Pain commonly radiates from the oropharynx toward the ear
Postherpetic neuralgia[12–14]	• Occurs after an acute episode of herpes zoster • Constant or intermittent burning pain • Allodynia • Unilateral • Can occur months to years after resolution of an initial outbreak
Traumatic neuralgia/neuritis[15]	• Clear precipitating traumatic event (eg, extraction, bone graft, tissue graft, root canal, fracture) to a nerve in the affected area
Burning mouth syndrome[16]	• Spontaneous onset • Continuous burning of the tongue, palate, gingiva, lips, and/or pharynx (tongue is the most common location) • More common in women • Bilateral and symmetric • Not associated with systemic or local pathology • Occasional taste changes
Atypical odontalgia and phantom tooth pain[17,18]	• Persistent localized pain in a tooth or area of a missing/extracted tooth • Not associated with a systemic or local pathology • Moderate severity • Onset can coincide with dental treatment • Touching area can trigger more intense pain • Unnecessary dental treatment (eg, endodontic treatment, extractions) often performed without relief of pain
Atypical facial pain/persistent idiopathic facial pain[19]	• Long duration, lasting most of the day (if not continuous) • Unilateral, and is without autonomic signs or symptoms • Often in the nasolabial fold or side of the chin • Psychological symptoms often present • Symptoms do not meet diagnostic criteria of other facial pain syndromes • Treatment is typically less effective than that of other facial pain syndromes, and a multidisciplinary approach is required to address the many facets of this condition

causing diffuse tooth pain that cannot be easily localized), but on many occasions it is directly caused by disease of the oral cavity associated with the following structures

- ○ Dentition (eg, dentin sensitivity, caries, pulpal disease)
- ○ Periodontium (eg, gingivitis, acute or chronic periodontal disease, sensitivity related to recession, or alveolar bone pathology)

- ○ Other soft and hard tissues including the palate, floor of mouth, buccal mucosa, nontooth-supporting bone, and tongue (caused by mucosal diseases, neoplasms, or pain related to parafunction or trauma)
- ○ Atypical odontalgia (described in the section on neuropathic pain)

It often is easy to rule out pain related to a specific area or structure in the oral cavity, since the pain is reproducible upon manipulation (eg, percussion, palpation, heat or cold testing, air) of the previously mentioned structures. Additionally, radiographs can assist in confirming or discounting the clinician's hypothesis. Classic signs of pulpal pain include sharp pain related to a specific tooth; periodontal pain is in general dull and throbbing, and pathology of the other soft tissues or underlying bone can present in a variety of ways. As previously discussed, intraoral pain can also refer to nearby anatomic structures (eg, a toothache causing an earache or headache). Clinicians with a dental background may not overlook such occurrences; however, it is important that those without dental training refer patients if they suspect pain is related to the dentition or its associated structures.

In general, a clinician may not view intraoral pain as something serious, but it is important not to disregard more severe etiologies that are less common. A thorough history of present illness and past medical history can usually assist in making these diagnoses (**Table 3**).

Temporomandibular Disorder

Temporomandibular disorder is a common complaint of orofacial pain and is defined as pain related to the[1,20] temporomandibular joint and muscles of mastication (masseter, temporalis, digastric, medial pterygoid, lateral pterygoid) or other muscles of the head and neck region.

When including temporomandibular disorder as a potential diagnosis, a thorough facial pain examination can usually elicit whether pain is related to the joint, muscles, or a combination of both. Muscular problems are usually reproducible upon palpation or resistance against active muscle movement. Joint problems (eg, disc displacement with or without reduction, capsulitis, synovitis, arthritis, or retrodiscitis) can also be detected through similar measures, and with the use of radiographs if necessary. These imaging modalities can vary from a simple panoramic radiograph, to a computed tomography scan, or magnetic resonance imaging (MRI) when applicable. A functional MRI can be useful for a real-time view of the anatomic structures during joint movement.

Additionally, one must consider that if a patient has generalized muscle pain and/or arthritis, temporomandibular disorder could be the manifestation of this underlying cause of systemic pain (**Table 4**).

Cervical Pain

Anatomically, the cervical area is the base and supporting structure of the head and neck region.[1] Because of their proximity and common nerve pathways, cervical spine disorders (CSDs) can refer pain to the orofacial region. Barring referred pain, a thorough examination should include the cervical area, its muscles, and bony components. This can be accomplished through palpation and also assessing the patient's neck movement—rotation, flexion, extensions, and side-to-side movements. If a CSD is suspected, possibilities to include on the differential include

- ○ Myalgia of the cervical muscles
- ○ Disorders of the cervical spine (including a herniated discs, degenerative disc disease, osteoarthritis, fracture, and compression of the spinal column)

Table 3
Differential diagnosis of intraoral pain

Condition	Signs and Symptoms
Dental caries	• Decay present clinically and on radiograph • If extending to the pulp, can lead to more severe sharp, shooting pain
Dental abscess	• Possible periapical radiolucency noted on radiograph • Carious or periodontal defect noted • Possible swelling and/or purulence in adjacent soft tissues
Cracked tooth	• History of parafunction • Large restoration present • Presence of craze lines • Pain on release and biting
Sensitivity	• Galvanic effects due to proximity of metal restorations • Can occur postoperatively after a restoration due to proximity to the pulp or leakage between the tooth and restoration seal • Presence of dentin exposure or root exposure
Premature bite/occlusal interferences	• Clear marking of an occlusal discrepancy with articulating paper • Resolution with adjustment
Dry socket	• 1–3 d after extraction • Loss of blood clot • Limited relief with conventional pain medication
Periodontal (gingivitis and periodontitis)	• Gingival erythema and/or edema with possible bleeding • Poor hygiene • Accumulation of plaque and calculus • Presence of deep periodontal pockets • Horizontal or vertical bone loss noted on radiograph • Pain is in general more dull and throbbing • Pain sometimes correlates with amount of stimulus
Pericoronitis	• Inflamed tissue surrounding an unerupted third molar
Mucosal pain	• Presence of vesiculoerosive conditions (eg, lichen planus, pemphigoid, pemphigus), soft tissue pathology, infection, trauma, xerostomia/dry mouth

Similar to many of the previously listed possibilities on a differential diagnosis, there can be a combination of a referred component and a local component.

Pain Related to Associated Structures

The complexity of head and neck anatomy and the amount of vital structures encompassed should encourage the practitioner to have a working knowledge of these structures, their function, and how they could possibly contribute to orofacial pain.[1] These areas include, but are not limited to

- Eyes
- Sinus cavities
- Ears
- Throat
- Nose
- Lymph nodes
- Salivary glands
- Vasculature

Table 4
Differential diagnosis of temporomandibular disorder

Condition	Signs and Symptoms
Myofascial pain and local myalgia	• Regional pain of masticatory muscles or muscles of the head and neck on palpation • Fatigue or tightness present • Pain is usually dull, throbbing, and/or aching • Aggravated by function and/or overuse • Possible presence of trigger points or tight bands of muscle • Myospasm of muscles of mastication can cause decreased opening • If chronic, can be more diffuse and centrally mediated
Disc displacement with reduction	• Clicking or popping of the affected side • Not necessarily painful • If unilateral, deviation to the affected side on opening • Usually no limitation of maximal opening
Disc displacement without reduction	• Functional impairment caused by limited opening/locking • If unilateral, deflection to affected side on opening • Clear displacement of the disc on imaging studies • Limitation of maximal opening
Temporomandibular joint dislocation	• Open lock • Condyle positioned anterior to the articular eminence • May require clinician manipulation for reduction
Osteoarthritis/degenerative joint disease	• Pain on palpation of the joint and during function • Adaptive changes (eg, condylar flattening, osteophytic changes) seen on imaging studies • If unilateral, deviation to affected side on opening • Possible limitation in opening • Crepitus present • Can be secondary to another disease or trauma
Capsulitis/synovitis/retrodiscitis	• Localized pain of the affected joint that is exacerbated by function • Can cause difficulty occluding on the posterior teeth of the affected side • Limited (if any) osteoarthritic changes noted on imaging studies

Similar to their surrounding anatomy, these structures can cause pain locally or via referral patterns. A thorough examination, including testing of cranial nerves, can assist in determining if one the previously mentioned structures is the primary etiology of pain. If a problem is suspected beyond the scope of one's practice or knowledge, then the patient should be referred appropriately.

Referred Pain

Referred pain has been discussed in some of the previous sections. It is important to take into account referred pain as a possibility when no abnormal findings are seen locally in the symptomatic location.

Psychiatric or Mental Illness

When evaluating an orofacial pain patient, conduct of a brief yet thorough psychological or psychiatric evaluation should always be performed, especially if the pain is chronic in nature.[1,20] Many psychiatric and emotional conditions (eg, depression, anxiety, chronic stress) can directly lead to pain secondary to parafunctional habits, sleep disturbances, and via upregulation of the autonomic nervous system. Subsequently, pain can exacerbate the original precipitating factor, and vice versa, thus creating a cycle that is difficult to break.

Another issue that must be dealt with when evaluating a patient with a comorbid mental condition is appropriate setting of expectations. Many of these patients have been to multiple providers and have been given a variety of treatment modalities. It is important to bring these patients' expectation sto a realistic level, which usually means possible improvement of their pain, but not necessarily resolution.

It is also important to note that having a mental illness does not imply that the psychiatric condition is the etiology of the orofacial pain condition, as the two could be exclusive of each other. Additionally, chronic facial pain could be the underlying etiology of the psychiatric condition. Symptom and pharmacologic management of a patient in conjunction with a mental health professional is appropriate when indicated.

SUMMARY

Orofacial pain is a common complaint of patients seen by dental professionals. Even if this complaint is not the primary reason for a patient seeking treatment, or the pain is nonodontogenic in origin, it is still important to acknowledge the problem to find an appropriate route to proceed. Whether this involves treatment of the condition or referral to another practitioner for assessment, formulating an inclusive differential diagnosis is a crucial step in the process. A broad range of possibilities prevents the provider from making a diagnosis too quickly, and most importantly assures that more serious causes are not overlooked or mistaken for common, less-threatening conditions.

REFERENCES

1. De Leeuw R. Orofacial pain: guidelines for assessment, diagnosis, and management. 4th edition. Hanover Park (IL): Quintessence Publishing Co, Inc; 2008.
2. Kelman L. The premonitory symptoms (prodrome): a tertiary care study of 893 migraineurs. Headache 2004;44:865.
3. Cutrer FM, Huerter K. Migraine aura. Neurologist 2007;13:118.
4. Manzoni GC, Terzano MG, Bono G, et al. Cluster headache—clinical findings in 180 patients. Cephalalgia 1983;3:21.
5. Drummond PD. Dysfunction of the sympathetic nervous system in cluster headache. Cephalalgia 1988;8:181.
6. Drummond PD. Mechanisms of autonomic disturbance in the face during and between attacks of cluster headache. Cephalalgia 2006;26:633.
7. Spierings EL, Ranke AH, Honkoop PC. Precipitating and aggravating factors of migraine versus tension-type headache. Headache 2001;41:554.
8. Cittadini E, Matharu MS, Goadsby PJ. Paroxysmal hemicrania: a prospective clinical study of 31 cases. Brain 2008;131:1142.
9. Hunder GG, Bloch DA, Michel BA, et al. The American College of Rheumatology 1990 criteria for the classification of giant cell arteritis. Arthritis Rheum 1990; 33(8):1122.
10. Headache Classification Subcommittee of the International Headache Society. The international classification of headache disorders: 2nd edition. Cephalalgia 2004;24(Suppl 1):9.

11. Rozen TD. Trigeminal neuralgia and glossopharyngeal neuralgia. Neurol Clin 2004;22:185.
12. Dworkin RH, Portenoy RK. Pain and its persistence in herpes zoster. Pain 1996; 67:241.
13. Bowsher D. Pathophysiology of postherpetic neuralgia: towards a rational treatment. Neurology 1995;45:S56.
14. Schott GD. Triggering of delayed-onset postherpetic neuralgia. Lancet 1998;351: 419.
15. Lewis MA, Sankar V, De Laat A, et al. Management of neuropathic orofacial pain. Oral Surg Oral Med Oral Pathol Oral Radiol Endod 2007;103(Suppl):S32.e1–24.
16. Patton LL, Siegel MA, Benoliel R, et al. Management of burning mouth syndrome: systematic review and management recommendations. Oral Surg Oral Med Oral Pathol Oral Radiol Endod 2007;103(Suppl):S39.e1–13.
17. Badd-Hansen L. Atypical odontalgia - pathophysiology and clinical management. J Oral Rehabil 2008;35(1):1–11.
18. Abiko Y, Matsuoka H, Chiba I, et al. Current evidence on atypical odontalgia: diagnosis and clinical management. Int J Dent 2012;2012:518548.
19. Agostoni E, Frigerio R, Santoro P. Atypical facial pain: clinical considerations and differential diagnosis. Neurol Sci 2005;26:S71–4.
20. Zakrzewska J. Orofacial pain. New York: Oxford University Press, Inc; 2008.

Intraoral Pain Disorders

Joel J. Napeñas, DDS[a,b,*]

KEYWORDS

- Caries • Pulpitis • Cracked tooth syndrome • Periapical disease • Alveolar osteitis
- Candidiasis

KEY POINTS

- Dental and pulpal pains are variable in their behavior, can refer to other structures distant from the source, and can mimic other facial pain disorders. Therefore it is essential that all complaints of pain in the mouth and face include ruling out pain of dental origin.
- Periodontal pain is more localizable than pulpal pain, usually by placing pressure apically or laterally on the involved tooth, or through the presence of identifiable clinical abnormality.
- Oral mucosal pain is a superficial somatic pain that is localizable, with the site and source common, and is responsive to local anesthesia in the affected area.
- Pain originating from the bone is due to inflammatory disorders from infection or injury. The severity of pain is related to the degree of confinement of exudate or purulence within the anatomic sites.

INTRODUCTION

Dental and oral diseases are common findings in the general population. Pain associated with dental caries or periodontal disease is the primary reason why most patients seek treatment from dental providers. Many patients who present with a complaint of oral pain have irrefutable clinical decay (**Fig. 1**). However, intraoral pain is not exclusively a result of dental disorders.

This review outlines common somatic intraoral pain disorders, which can originate from disease involving 1 or more broad anatomic areas, the teeth, the surrounding soft tissues (mucogingival, tongue, salivary glands), and bone.

DENTAL AND PULPAL

When examining pain of dental origin, one must determine if is related to the teeth or pulp directly, or if it is due to irritation of the surrounding periodontal ligament. There is

The author has nothing to disclose.
[a] Division of Oral Medicine and Radiology, Schulich School of Medicine and Dentistry, Dental Sciences Building, Western University, London, ON N6A 5C1, Canada; [b] Department of Oral Medicine, Carolinas Medical Center, PO Box 32861, Charlotte, NC 28232, USA
* Division of Oral Medicine and Radiology, Schulich School of Medicine and Dentistry, Dental Sciences Building, Western University, London, ON N6A 5C1, Canada.
E-mail address: joel.napenas@schulich.uwo.ca

Dent Clin N Am 57 (2013) 429–447
http://dx.doi.org/10.1016/j.cden.2013.04.004
0011-8532/13/$ – see front matter © 2013 Elsevier Inc. All rights reserved.

dental.theclinics.com

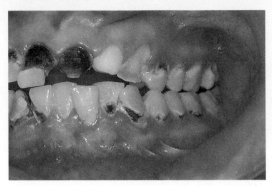

Fig. 1. Rampant caries caused by impaired function of salivary gland.

a continuum of pain symptoms that are based on the degree or severity of disease. This continuum ranges from the short, sharp, localizable pain, a physiologic response or warning of noxious stimuli or impending pathologic state, and progresses to the persistent, dull pain that indicates the presence of inflammation, infection, and disease.

Dental and pulpal pain occurs when there is noxious stimulation of the teeth and/or disease affecting the enamel, dentin, or pulpal structures. The disease involves breach of tooth structure attributable to mechanical means (eg, trauma, attrition, abrasion, erosion, iatrogenic) and/or bacteria (ie, caries).

Enamel is avascular, noninnervated, and nonporous, therefore demineralization of or the presence of caries isolated in the enamel is usually painless. Once lesions breach the dentinoenamel junction, pain is experienced through stimuli affecting the dentinal tubules. Myelinated (Aδ) and unmyelinated (C) fibers innervate the pulp. If there is sufficient stimulation (eg, via heat, cold, or pressure), fluid movement in the dentinal tubules activates the low-threshold Aδ fibers, producing the quick, sharp, localized pain. An injured tooth with local inflammation lowers the pain threshold of Aδ fibers. Once there is pulpal involvement and inflammation persists the C fibers are stimulated, producing a more prolonged, dull, and diffuse pain.

A tooth causing pain is initially identified by obtaining a history from the patient, then identifying a tooth with clinical evidence of abnormality (eg, fracture, caries, lost restoration, abrasion). An attempt is then made to increase the pain through noxious stimulation of the tooth in question via mechanical (eg, percussion, biting), thermal (eg, cold and heat), electric (eg, electric pulp testing [EPT]), or chemical means. Radiographs can then be taken of the teeth to for pathologic evaluation.

Caries

Caries occurs through bacterial invasion of the tooth structures, resulting in decay caused by formation of acid metabolites. It may occur on enamel, dentin, and cementum on exposed root surfaces. Patients may complain of thermal sensitivity or sensitivity when exposed to sweet or acidic foods. Pain is sharp, localized, and dissipates immediately after removal of the stimuli. Sensitivity derives from lost enamel and increased exposure of dentin and cementum.

Caries is detected and diagnosed both clinically and radiographically (**Fig. 2**). Management of dental caries varies by the size of the lesion as well as the state of the caries. If a lesion is incipient, monitoring and/or topical fluoride placement is adequate. However, if the lesion extends into dentin and is not arrested, removal of the decayed tooth structure and placement of a dental restoration may be required.

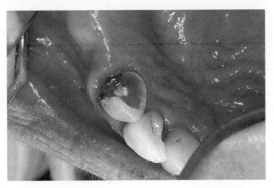

Fig. 2. Carious tooth.

Exposed Cementum or Dentin

Exposed cementum or dentin is most commonly caused by incorrect tooth-brushing technique resulting in gingival recession and/or abrasion of enamel (**Fig. 3**). Tooth sensitivity to cold liquids generally results. Pain is also sharp, localized, and dissipates immediately after removal of the cold stimuli. Treatment measures are directed toward limiting dentinal fluid movement by covering the exposed dentin or cementum, which is achieved with oral hygiene instructions to improve tooth-brushing technique, use of desensitizing agents, and sometimes restorations.[1,2]

Pulpal Disease

The most common cause of pulpal pain is dental caries that extends to the pulp; however, other causes include trauma, fracture, exposed dentin or cementum, or premature contact. Acute pulpal pain acts like other visceral type pains, with diffuseness and variability. There may be continuous dull, aching pain with superimposed episodes of pulsing, throbbing, and sharp pain, representing stimulation of the C fibers and the lower threshold of $A\delta$ fibers, respectively. Pulpal pain can be modified by a variety of stimuli including heat, cold, pressure, and head positioning. Teeth that only have pulpal disease are not sensitive to percussion. The specific features of and management strategies for various pulpal disease states are as follows:

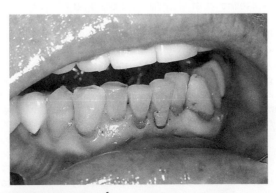

Fig. 3. Exposed cementum on root surfaces.

Normal

Normal pulp has a short response to cold stimuli that subsides almost immediately on removal. There is no evidence of periapical abnormality on radiographs. In the absence of tooth abnormality, no treatment is indicated.

Reversible pulpitis

Reversible pulpitis is characterized by an exaggerated quick, sharp response to cold stimuli, followed by a dull ache that dissipates. There is no complaint of spontaneous pain. Tooth is not tender to percussion, and there is no radiographic evidence of periapical abnormality. Treatment of reversible pulpitis entails removal of the pain-causing stimulus, usually removal of lesion, and restoration of lost tooth structure, as it does not require extirpation of the pulp through root canal therapy (RCT) or extraction of the tooth.

Irreversible pulpitis

Irreversible pulpitis presents as spontaneous, lingering dull ache or constant severe, unrelenting pain; increased pain intensity to noxious stimuli; and positive response to cold and heat stimuli (ie, sharp response followed by dull ache that persists.) Radiographically there may or may not be a thickening in the periodontal ligament (PDL) at the tooth's apex. Treatment requires either RCT or tooth extraction.

Pulpal necrosis

In pulpal necrosis there is no pain and no response to noxious stimuli (cold, heat, or EPT). Radiographs may or may not reveal the presence of a periapical radiolucency. If the infection has extended beyond the apex of the tooth into the surrounding bone (see the section on acute apical periodontitis), a percussion test may be positive. Treatment requires either RCT or extraction.

Cracked Tooth Syndrome

Cracked tooth is defined as incomplete fracture of the dentin that may or may not extend to the pulp.[3] The term cracked tooth syndrome was first introduced by Cameron in 1964, describing when the fractures become symptomatic.[4]

Patient complaints include sharp, momentary pain that is stimulated by biting or releasing, or resulting from exposure to cold food or drinks. The pain in cracked tooth syndrome can be easily localized.[4] Pain sometimes may linger minutes after chewing.[5]

Diagnosis is often difficult because of the lack of clinical and radiographic findings. It is determined through careful history taking and clinical examination. Visual inspection of the tooth should be performed. Tactile inspection with an explorer tip may also be performed. Radiographs should be reviewed with bitewings preferred over periapical films; however, the likelihood of visualizing a cracked tooth on a radiograph is rare (**Fig. 4**). A useful diagnostic aid is transillumination, best performed with use of magnification to better illustrate color changes and clinically significant cracks. Tooth percussion should be performed; however, pain is seldom elicited with percussion in the apical direction. Pain on biting may be noted, but is more commonly noted with release of biting, owing to fluids within dentinal tubules moving toward the pulp.[5]

Treatment of cracked tooth syndrome may include stabilization with an orthodontic band or more permanently with a crown or overlay, or with RCT or extraction of the tooth depending on the extent of the crack.

PERIODONTAL

Periodontal pain (eg, periodontium and alveolar bone) is more localized than pulpal pain, owing to the proprioceptors and mechanoreceptors in the periodontium.[6] Pain

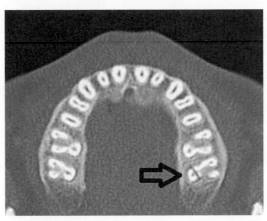

Fig. 4. Fractured palatal root of upper left second molar (*arrow*), as seen on an axial-view computed tomography (CT) image.

caused by chronic periodontal conditions (eg, gingivitis, chronic periodontitis) is generally nonexistent, or may be mild, persistent, or episodic dull pain attributable to inflammation or low-grade infection.

Periodontal pain caused by local factors is localized to affected teeth in which there is inflammation or infection involving the gingiva, periodontium, alveolar bone, or pericoronal tissue. Bacterial infection is usually the causative factor. The bulk of the discussion in this section is focused on these conditions.

Gingival/Periodontal Abscess

Gingival abscesses are relatively uncommon, whereas periodontal abscesses are more common and occur in areas of periodontal disease. Pain complaints can range from low-intensity aches to severe, sharp pain. Pain is made worse by chewing and percussion of adjacent teeth.

Gingival abscesses are confined to the marginal interdental tissue. Both show localized swelling of the gingiva, which may also include alveolar mucosa. Lesions are fluctuant, violacious, and cyanotic or erythematous in appearance, and may or may not be accompanied by drainage via fistula.[7]

Abscesses are caused by the proliferation of periodontal bacterial flora in a diseased periodontal site, although they can also be caused by food or foreign-body impaction or trauma. Abscess microflora contains mostly periodontal pathogens, including *Porphyromonas gingivalis*, *Prevotella intermedia*, *Fusobacterium nucleatum*, *Peptostreptococcus micros* and *Bacterioides forsythus*.[8]

Areas of periodontal disease involve tissue destruction (connective tissue and bone) caused by activation of host inflammatory mediators in response to bacterial microorganisms. The abscess is a focus of purulent exudate in connective tissue, surrounded by infiltration of leukocytes, edematous tissue, and vessels.

Clinical features as described, in conjunction with clinical evidence (eg, deep pockets, horizontal bone loss, gingival edema, and/or erythema) and radiographic evidence of periodontal disease, are sufficient to obtain a diagnosis of a periodontal abscess. Clinical features in the absence of periodontal disease, and a history of trauma, support the diagnosis of a gingival abscess (**Fig. 5**).

Treatment of the abscess entails obtaining purulent drainage, either by incision of the fluctuant area or through the pocket orifice. This action is accompanied by removal

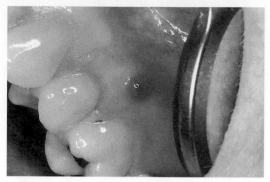

Fig. 5. Gingival abscess on upper left maxillary gingiva.

of the causative agent (eg, foreign body or bacterial foci). Root debridement is performed for periodontal abscesses.

Periapical Disease

Patient complaints include a rapid onset of moderate to severe spontaneous pain that is sharp, throbbing, or aching in nature, pain to percussion of affected teeth, purulence, and/or swelling (**Fig. 6**). Pain is more severe if the abscess is confined to bone; however, if it finds a path into soft tissues and forms a fluctuant pus-filled swelling or a fistula, it can decrease. In more long-standing and chronic cases there may not be any complaints of pain, or only the presence of mild discomfort.

Periapical disease occurs when a bacterial infection of necrotic pulp spreads into the periapical tissues. Virulent bacteria infiltrate the apical PDL, leading to an acute inflammatory reaction.

Diagnostic steps are the same as those outlined for pulpal disease (see earlier discussion). Through clinical examination it must be established that the tooth is nonvital with a necrotic pulp. Periapical diagnoses can be classified as follows.

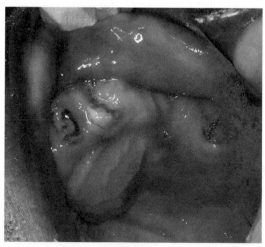

Fig. 6. Abscess on the upper right palate associated with necrotic teeth.

Normal
There is no response to percussion or palpation. Radiographic findings are normal, with intact lamina dura (LD) and uniform PDL space.

Acute (symptomatic) apical periodontitis
This condition is characterized by a complaint of spontaneous pain (moderate to severe). Clinical findings include a nonvital tooth, pain on percussion, and biting of the affected tooth. Radiographs may show widened PDL space and intact LD (**Fig. 7**).

Asymptomatic apical periodontitis
The affected tooth is established as nonvital (eg, no response to cold or EPT) and there is an unremarkable response to percussion or palpation. Radiographic findings include a break in LD, widening PDL space, or the presence of a periapical radiolucency (PARL) (**Fig. 8**).

Acute apical abscess
Acute apical abscess is characterized by a rapid onset of spontaneous pain and swelling of the gingival and alveolar mucosa (unless abscess is confined to bone). Radiographs may or may not show periapical changes.

Chronic apical abscess
This condition is a long-standing focus of infection, usually with little or no discomfort, caused by a path of drainage with a fistula or sinus tract.

Management of periapical disease requires treating the affected tooth via RCT or extraction. If the abscess involves an area of fluctuant swelling, incision and drainage may also be required.

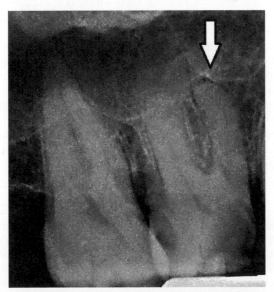

Fig. 7. Widened periodontal ligament at the apex of the distal root (*arrow*) of a carious maxillary first molar. (*Courtesy of* Nader S. Jahshan, DDS, Brantford, Ontario, Canada.)

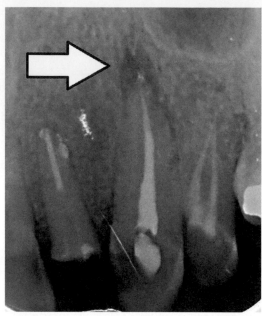

Fig. 8. Periapical radiolucency (*arrow*) on root canal treated upper left canine. (*Courtesy of* Nader S. Jahshan DDS, Brantford, Ontario, Canada.)

Alveolar Osteitis (Dry Socket)

This condition occurs 1 to 5 days after a tooth extraction, and is described by patients as a moderate to severe, deep, continuous, aching, radiating pain that originates in the area of the tooth extraction but may be difficult to localize. It is only partially relieved by analgesic medications. There is an absence of swelling or purulence. Examination of the extraction site reveals exposed bare bone in the tooth socket, which is very sensitive to probing and may emit a foul odor.

Alveolar osteitis occurs when the blood clot in the socket is lost through mechanical means (eg, excessive rinsing or spitting), smoking, or possibly fibrinolytic components in saliva. Thus bare alveolar bone in the socket is exposed to bacteria and food debris, and resultant inflammation and/or infection occurs.

A history of recent tooth extraction, combined with the clinical features, is sufficient to determine a diagnosis.

Treatment entails irrigation and cleansing of the socket to remove bacteria and debris, and application of a topical medicament into the socket to provide analgesia (ie, by cauterizing exposed nerve endings) and antiseptic effects; this is accompanied by more potent oral analgesics for pain.

Periocoronitis

Pericoronitis is inflammation and localized infection of tissue structures surrounding the crown of an impacted tooth, which frequently occurs in the area of fully or partially impacted third molars. Pain is usually continuous, ranges from mild to severe, and can be described as aching, throbbing, and/or sharp, radiating to the ear, throat, and floor of mouth. An erythematous and edematous gingival lesion is seen, and indentation of the opposing tooth is seen frequently. Swelling, purulent discharge, and lymphadenopathy may also be present.

Bacterial growth occurs in the space between the crown of the tooth and the overlying gingival tissue, which may be due to food impaction, trauma (owing to opposing dentition), or inability to clean the site.

Clinical features and the presence of an impacted tooth are sufficient to obtain a diagnosis, which may also be confirmed with radiographs.

Antibiotic therapy is appropriate for proper management. A more conservative approach may involve removal of the operculum overlying the affected tooth; however, hygiene and soft-tissue management in this area is difficult. For prevention, ultimate treatment involves extraction of the affected tooth as well as the tooth in the opposing arch.

ORAL MUCOSAL PAIN

Oral pain related to mucosal disorders is a direct manifestation of changes of the mucosal epithelium. These changes are seen intraorally as vesicle formation, ulcerations, erosions, erythema, pseudomembranes, and/or hyperkeratosis, with hyperalgesia of the affected mucosal tissue.

Pain of mucosal origin is continuous; usually described as raw, stinging, aching, and burning; can be reliably provoked by exposure to stimuli (thermal, mechanical, and chemical); and usually responds to the application of topical or local anesthetic at the site of pain.

Painful oral mucosal disorders may develop as a result of infection (bacterial, viral, or fungal), reactive processes (trauma, allergy, iatrogenic), systemic disorders (autoimmune or metabolic), or dysplasia (cancer). A comprehensive review of mucogingival diseases is beyond the scope of this review; however, select notable and common conditions are briefly discussed.

Oral Candidiasis

Oral candidiasis represents inflammatory conditions caused by infection from the yeast fungi genus *Candida*. The most common cause of oral candidiasis is the species *Candida albicans*. Infection can occur because of change in bacterial flora from antibiotics, lack of saliva, or conditions that impair local or systemic immune function (eg, diabetes, human immunodeficiency virus [HIV]). Acute pseudomembranous candidiasis is the most common form, affecting any intraoral mucosal surface, presenting with superficial, curd-like, white plaques that can be wiped off, overlying an erythematous, eroded, or ulcerated surface (**Fig. 9**). Acute atrophic candidiasis is more painful, with red lesions surrounded by inflamed tissue, with symptoms including oral burning and dysphagia. Chronic atrophic candidiasis appears erythematous and edematous, with a papular surface. Lesions occur on edentulous ridges or palate, frequently under dentures. Chronic hyperplastic candidiasis results in white and/or red hard nodular lesions that cannot be wiped off.

Diagnosis is often made from history and clinical appearance. If a diagnosis is uncertain or the condition arises in immunocompromised patients, a cytologic smear and culture may be performed to identify specific organism.

Oral candidiasis can be addressed with topical medicaments including chlorhexidine rinse, nystatin rinse or ointment, or clotrimazole troches. In refractory cases or in the immunocompromised, systemic medications are used, which include fluconazole, ketoconazole, and itraconazole.

Herpes Simplex Virus

Herpes simplex virus (HSV) infection can cause an acute primary or recurrent oral infection through two different strains, HSV-1 and HSV-2. Primary herpetic

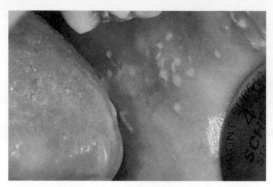

Fig. 9. Pseudomembranous candidiasis on the left buccal mucosa.

gingivostomatitis occurs in those who have not been previously exposed to the virus (eg, children or adolescents). It initially presents with a painful, severe, generalized gingival inflammation, followed by oral vesicles, accompanied by systemic manifestations including fever, malaise, and lymphadenopathy. After initial infection, which in most cases is subclinical, the virus remains latent or dormant within the trigeminal ganglion. Reactivation causes secondary or recurrent herpes stomatitis, which presents as painful vesicle eruptions, typically occurring on keratinized tissue (eg, lips, gingiva, tongue, hard palate) (**Fig. 10**). These eruptions may be preceded by prodromal tingling or burning sensations. Vesicles are quickly ruptured, resulting in a yellow ulceration with erythematous borders. Healing occurs within 1 to 4 days. Treatment of primary herpetic gingivostomatitis is supportive (fluids, nutrition, and analgesia). For recurrent herpes stomatitis, topical pencyclovir and oral valacyclovir (2 g twice a day for 1 day in the early prodromal stages) have been shown to decrease the severity and length of outbreak.[9,10] Other considerations include topical docosanol and oral acyclovir.

Herpes Zoster (Shingles)

Herpes zoster is an oral infection attributable to the varicella zoster virus, which causes chicken pox. Higher-risk individuals include the elderly and immunocompromised. The virus remains latent and dormant in nerve tissue, with the trigeminal

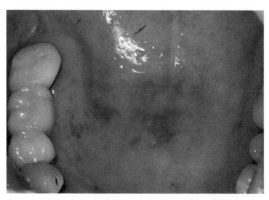

Fig. 10. Herpes simplex virus lesions on the hard palate. Ulcerations remain after bursting of vesicles.

ganglion involved in 10% to 15% of cases, among which 80% involves the ophthalmic division (V1).[11] It is characterized by prodromal symptoms of pain, burning, and tingling, followed by vesicular eruption, rupture, and ulceration in the distribution of the trigeminal nerve within 1 week of onset (**Fig. 11**). Eruptions can be seen both intra-orally and extraorally on the skin. Diagnosis is made by history and clinical presentation. Treatment involves systemic antivirals such as acyclovir, valacyclovir, and famciclovir, accompanied by analgesics. Oral corticosteroids are also used to decrease the severity and duration of pain.[12] The most common complication of herpes zoster is post-herpetic neuralgia, a neuropathic condition causing continuous intractable pain that is burning and aching in nature.

Necrotizing Periodontal Disease

Necrotizing periodontal disease encompasses both necrotizing ulcerative gingivitis (NUG) and necrotizing ulcerative periodontitis (NUP). Although the exact etiology is unknown, spirochetes and fusiform bacteria are implicated, and factors include stress, tobacco use, poor oral hygiene, and impaired immunity. The condition presents as a continuously painful, erythematous, and edematous gingiva with punched-out erosion of the interdental papilla, often covered with a gray necrotic pseudomembrane. A fetid odor is common, and systemic symptoms (eg, malaise, low-grade fever) may be present. Diagnosis is obtained through history and clinical symptoms. Treatment consists of mechanical debridement, antibiotic therapy (chlorhexidine rinse, metronidazole, tetracycline, doxycycline), and management of underlying periodontal disease.

Recurrent Aphthous Stomatitis

Recurrent aphthous stomatitis (RAS) is the most common ulcerative condition of the oral cavity.[13] Ulcers most commonly occur in nonkeratinized mucosa (eg, lips, labial and buccal mucosa, ventral tongue, floor of mouth, and soft palate). Pain is continuous and is described as burning and aching, with pain that is disproportionate to the size of the lesions. Lesions can appear solitary or multiple, showing as a yellow ulceration with erythematous border (**Fig. 12**). The exact etiology of RAS is unknown; however, precipitating factors include certain foods, trauma, stress, hormones, nutritional or hematinic deficiencies, and contents of oral hygiene products.[14] Diagnosis is generally elicited by history and clinical presentations, and may include attempts to identify any underlying causes, which may entail history of foods and oral care products as well as blood work. Lesions typically last for 7 to 10 days, followed by complete

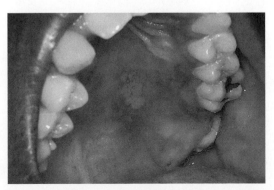

Fig. 11. Herpes zoster lesions on the left hard palate. Lesions are unilateral, following the distribution of the second branch of the trigeminal nerve (V2).

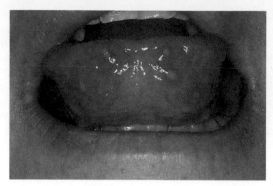

Fig. 12. Recurrent aphthous stomatitis. Multiple ulcerations on the ventral tongue.

healing. Treatment is based on palliation, with topical anesthetics as an option.[15] Other topical agents, primarily aimed at curbing inflammation, include topical tetracyclines and chlorhexidine rinse. Topical steroids are used to possibly decrease the length and severity of symptoms.[16] In refractory, recurrent, and more severe cases, or in the immunocompromised (eg, HIV), systemic immune modulators such as oral corticosteroids, dapsone, pentoxifylline, and thalidomide are used.

Lichen Planus

Lichen planus is a dermatologic disease that often affects the oral mucosa. There are two forms: reticular lichen planus, which is most often asymptomatic, and erosive lichen planus, which is the type more likely to be symptomatic and characterized by burning, or pain when eating or drinking. Reticular lichen planus often shows white lines or striae (often in a reticular or lace-like pattern), or plaques or papules, overlying an area of erythema. Erosive lichen planus is characterized by erythematous areas with ulceration, usually bordered by white striae (**Fig. 13**). Affected areas are the buccal mucosa, tongue, gingiva, palate, and vermillion border. The characteristic reticular pattern is enough of a clinical presentation to obtain a diagnosis; however, biopsy may be required to obtain a diagnosis through histopathologic confirmation. Treatment is indicated only if the patient is symptomatic, and usually consists of

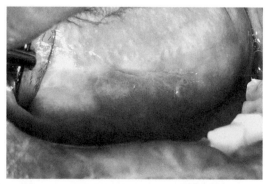

Fig. 13. Erosive lichen planus. Area of erythematous ulceration on the left lateral tongue, surrounded by white plaque and striae.

topical corticosteroids. Other considerations include topical tacrolimus or cyclosporine, or intralesional steroid injections in refractory areas.

Immunobullous Diseases

The immunobullous diseases include pemphigus vulgaris (PV) and mucous membrane pemphigoid (MMP), also known as cicatricial pemphigoid. Autoantibodies cause damage to the epithelium and underlying connective tissue. Patients' chief complaint is continuous oral soreness in affected areas. Clinical presentation of both includes vesicles, erosions, and ulceration in the oral mucosa and skin, with oral manifestations often being the first symptom to appear (**Figs. 14** and **15**). MMP also can affect the eyes, esophagus, and laryngeal and vaginal mucosa. Diagnosis is obtained through biopsy of both lesional and perilesional tissue, with the latter being used for staining for autoantibodies through direct immunofluorescence. In addition, patients' serum is collected to perform an indirect immunofluorescence analysis. MMP can be responsive to potent topical steroid therapy. Treatment of PV or refractory MMP involves systemic corticosteroids and other systemic immune modulators.

Cancer

Orofacial pain may be induced by malignant disease and its therapy. Pain has been reported in at least 50% of patients before, during, and at the end of cancer therapy, some persisting up to 1 year after the completion of therapy.[17]

Squamous cell carcinoma comprises 90% of intraoral malignancies, which in turn comprise 5% of all malignancies in the United States.[18] Pain from intraoral cancers can be due to long-standing ulcerations (**Fig. 16**), secondary infection, stimulation of nerve endings, or infiltration into adjacent peripheral nerve. Pain may be accompanied by paresthesia or hypoesthesia. Other clinical features include loose teeth, occlusal changes, bony expansion, and restricted jaw and/or tongue movement. Such symptoms must be viewed with high suspicion for malignancy when accompanied by pain, requiring further workup (eg, imaging studies, tissue biopsy) to obtain the correct diagnosis.

Oral Mucositis

Oral mucositis (OM) is a painful and debilitating side effect of cancer therapy, including chemotherapy, radiation therapy (to the head and neck), and hematopoietic stem cell transplantation for patients with hematologic malignancies. OM is characterized by erythema, ulceration, and pseudomembrane formation and shedding (**Fig. 17**). More

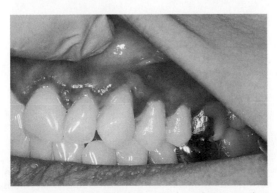

Fig. 14. Mucous membrane pemphigoid. Blisters and erythema on the maxillary gingiva.

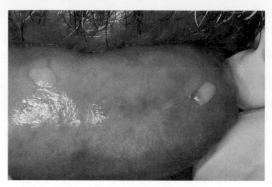

Fig. 15. Pemphigus vulgaris. Blisters on the labial mucosa.

than 40% of patients undergoing cancer chemotherapy contract some form of OM, and more than 60% develop a severe form of oral mucositis from radiation therapy and stem cell transplantation, with up to half of individuals requiring modification or interruption of their cancer treatment and/or parenteral analgesia.[19,20]

Treatment of OM is generally palliative with topical analgesic rinses, oral and parenteral analgesics, and supportive measures (eg, fluids, nutrition).

BONE
Osteomyelitis

Acute osteomyelitis occurs when an inflammatory process (usually infectious) spreads through the medullary spaces of the bone. Signs and symptoms include significant pain and sensitivity in the affected jaw area, swelling, fever, lymphadenopathy, and leukocytosis. This presentation may be accompanied by paresthesia, drainage, or exfoliation of bony sequestra. Chronic osteomyelitis may have swelling, pain, sinus formation, and periods of pain followed by remission. Diagnosis is obtained by combination of clinical symptoms and through imaging studies, which show ill-defined radiolucencies in the affected bone. Treatment entails drainage (in the presence of abscess formation) and antibiotic therapy. For refractory chronic osteomyelitis surgical intervention is required, involving removal of affected bone through curettage and, in more severe cases, resection.

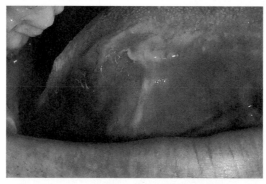

Fig. 16. Squamous cell carcinoma. Painful, nonhealing ulceration on the right lateral tongue that was confirmed as squamous cell carcinoma after biopsy and pathologic diagnosis.

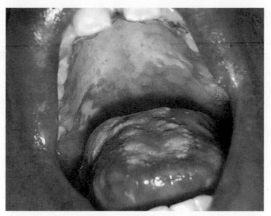

Fig. 17. Oral mucositis in a patient undergoing cancer chemotherapy.

Osteonecrosis

Osteonecrosis occurs because of hypoxia, hypovascularity, and hypocellularity of the bone. Osteoradionecrosis (ORN) and bisphosphonate osteonecrosis (BON) involve the formation of necrotic bone in the oral cavity in response to exposure to radiation therapy and bisphosphonate therapy, respectively. In addition, other, nonbisphosphonate drugs have been implicated in causing osteonecrosis. It is characterized by the presence of nonhealing area of exposed bone of at least 6 months' duration (**Fig. 18**).

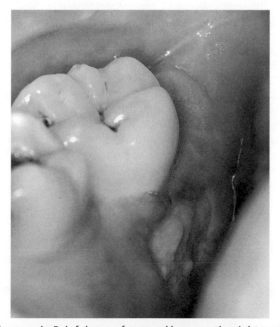

Fig. 18. Osteoradionecrosis. Painful area of exposed bone on the right posterior lingual area in a patient who had undergone radiation therapy to the head and neck.

Clinical manifestations and symptoms include pain, swelling, reduced jaw mobility, bony destruction, and purulent drainage when there is secondary osteomyelitis. Risk factors for ORN include radiation dosages higher than 60 Gy, dental disease, postradiation dental extractions, and previous cancer resection.[21] BON occurs in patients on oral bisphosphonates for osteoporosis; however those having been on intravenous bisphosphonate therapy for cancer involving the bone are at considerably higher risk and incidence.[22] Because of their nonhealing nature, treatment of both ORN and BON is challenging, and there is no established effective treatment regimen. Management strategies include analgesia, long-term topical and systemic antibiotic therapy for secondary infections, pentoxifylline, and hyperbaric oxygen therapy. Surgical considerations include removal of affected bone by curettage or resection and vascularized bone containing pedicle flap, although surgery may exacerbate the condition.

Maxillary Sinusitis

Toothache may be a presenting symptom of maxillary sinusitis, the most common causes of which are upper respiratory tract infection and allergic rhinitis.

Acute sinusitis
Clinical features include: headache; fever; facial pain over affected sinus; clear, mucoid, or purulent thick or thin anterior nasal or posterior pharyngeal discharge; pain over the cheekbone; toothache and tenderness to percussion of multiple maxillary teeth; periorbital pain; and pain during positional changes (increased pain when upright, decreased pain when supine).

Chronic sinusitis
Clinical features include: facial pressure and pain; sensation of obstruction, headache, and sore throat; lightheadedness; and generalized fatigue.

When normal (commensal) sinus flora is augmented, potential for infection is increased. Most common bacteria implicated are *Streptococcus pneumoniae* and *Haemophilus influenzae*. As the maxillary sinus is in close proximity to the maxillary posterior teeth, 10% of maxillary sinusitis cases may result from odontogenic sources, including infection or manipulation of posterior teeth.[23]

Clinical features, along with imaging studies (radiographs, computed tomography [CT], magnetic resonance imaging), aid in obtaining a diagnosis. Radiographically, increased radiopacities are seen in the sinus (**Fig. 19**).

Treatment is targeted at symptoms and includes decongestants, antihistamines, mucolytic agents, α-adrenergic agents, corticosteroids, and analgesics. Antibiotic

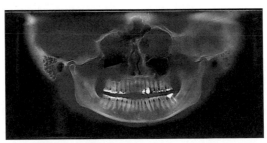

Fig. 19. Panoramic view of a CT image showing radio-opacities in the right maxillary sinus. (*Courtesy of* Richard H. Haug DDS, Charlotte, NC.)

use is indicated in cases of moderate to severe pain, persistence beyond 7 days, and purulent discharge.

SALIVARY GLAND ABNORMALITY
Bacterial Sialadenitis

Bacterial sialadenitis is a bacterial infection of the salivary gland. Clinical features include swollen and painful salivary glands, more often unilateral, with induration and erythema on the overlying skin. It most commonly occurs in patients with reduced salivary flow. Reduced salivary flow decreases mechanical flushing, leading to increased colonization of bacteria in the salivary gland ducts. Predominant bacterial species include *Staphylococcus aureus*, *H influenza*, *Streptococcus viridans*, *S pneumoniae*, *Escherichia coli*, and *Fusobacterium*, *Prevotella*, and *Porphyromonas* species.[24]

Oral Sialoliths

Oral sialoliths (salivary stones) are calcified material that forms within the major salivary glands. Most commonly they occur in the submandibular glands (80%–90%), followed by the parotid (5%–15%) and sublingual glands (2%–5%). Symptoms are based on the degree of obstruction of the duct and the presence of secondary infection. Pain may be accompanied by swelling and ulceration, and may be accompanied by fistulas and purulent drainage when secondary infection occurs. Radiographs (occlusal) and CT scans may show sialoliths; however, they are not always calcified enough to show up on these images (**Fig. 20**). Sialography and sialoendoscopy may also be used.

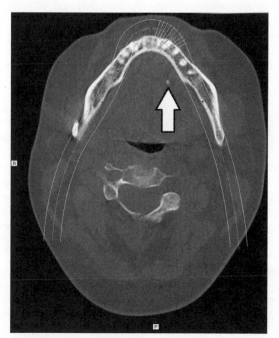

Fig. 20. Sialolith (*arrow*) seen on an axial-view CT image. (*Courtesy of* Richard H. Haug DDS, Charlotte, NC.)

Treatment in the acute phases for bacterial sialadenitis and sialoliths with secondary infection is mainly supportive, with use of analgesics, hydration, antibiotics, and para-sympathomimetics to stimulate salivary flow. For sialoliths, surgical removal of the salivary stone may also be indicated.

ACKNOWLEDGMENTS

Special thanks to Dawnyetta Marable, MD, DMD, for her significant contribution in the assembly of this article. Also a special mention to Andrea Herman, Leigha Christenbury Hernandez, and Katherine Tuori for their assistance.

REFERENCES

1. Orchardson R, Gillam DG. The efficacy of potassium salts as agents for treating dentin hypersensitivity. J Orofac Pain 2000;14(1):9–19.
2. Trowbridge HO, Silver DR. A review of current approaches to in-office management of tooth hypersensitivity. Dent Clin North Am 1990;34(3):561–81.
3. Mathew S, Thangavel B, Mathew CA, et al. Diagnosis of cracked tooth syndrome. J Pharm Bioallied Sci 2012;4(Suppl 2):S242–4.
4. Turp JC, Gobetti JP. The cracked tooth syndrome: an elusive diagnosis. J Am Dent Assoc 1996;127:1502–7.
5. Berman LH, Hartwell GR. Diagnosis. In: Cohen S, Hargreaves K, editors. Pathways of the pulp. 9th edition. St Louis (MO): Mosby; 2006. p. 1–39.
6. Van Steenberghe D. The structure and function of periodontal innervation. A review of the literature. J Periodontal Res 1979;14(3):185–203.
7. Abrams H, Jasper SJ. Diagnosis and management of acute periodontal problems. In: Falace DA, editor. Emergency dental care: diagnosis and management of urgent dental problems. Baltimore (MD): Williams & Wilkins; 1995. p. 137–42.
8. Herrera D, Roldan S, Gonzalez I, et al. The periodontal abscess. I. Clinical and microbiological findings. J Clin Periodontol 2000;27(6):387–94.
9. Spruance SL, Rea TL, Thoming C, et al. Penciclovir cream for the treatment of herpes simplex labialis. A randomized, multicenter, double-blind, placebo-controlled trial. Topical Penciclovir Collaborative Study Group. JAMA 1997; 277(17):1374–9.
10. Spruance SL, Jones TM, Blatter MM, et al. High-dose, short-duration, early vala-cyclovir therapy for episodic treatment of cold sores: results of two randomized, placebo-controlled, multicenter studies. Antimicrob Agents Chemother 2003;47: 1072–80.
11. Ragozzino MW, Melton LJ 3rd, Kurland LT, et al. Population-based study of herpes zoster and its sequelae. Medicine (Baltimore) 1982;61:310–6.
12. Eaglestein WH, Katz R, Brown JA. The effects of early corticosteroid therapy in the skin eruption and pain of herpes zoster. J Am Med Assoc 1970;211:1681–3.
13. Ship JA, Chavez EM, Doerr PA, et al. Recurrent aphthous stomatitis. Quintessence Int 2000;31:95–112.
14. Scully C, Gorsky M, Lozada-Nur F. The diagnosis and management of recurrent aphthous stomatitis: a consensus approach. J Am Dent Assoc 2003;134:200–7.
15. Eisen D, Lynch DP. Selecting topical and systemic agents for recurrent aphthous stomatitis. Cutis 2001;68:201–6.
16. Porter SR, Scully C, Pedersen A. Recurrent aphthous stomatitis. Crit Rev Oral Biol Med 1998;9(3):306–32.
17. Epstein JB, Hong C, Logan RM, et al. A systematic review of orofacial pain in patients receiving cancer therapy. Support Care Cancer 2010;18(8):1023–31.

18. Barasch A, Safford M, Eisenberg E. Oral cancer and oral effects of anticancer therapy. Mt Sinai J Med 1998;65(5–6):370–7.
19. Sonis ST. Oral complications. In: Holland JF, editor. Cancer medicine. 4th edition. Philadelphia: Williams & Wilkins; 1997. p. 3255–64.
20. Schubert MM, Sullivan KMJ, Truelove EL. Head and neck complication of bone marrow transplantation. Develop Oncol 1991;36:401–27.
21. Katsura K, Sasai K, Sato K, et al. Relationship between oral health status and development of osteoradionecrosis of the mandible: a retrospective longitudinal study. Oral Surg Oral Med Oral Pathol Oral Radiol Endod 2008;105:731–8.
22. Migliorati CA, Woo SB, Hewson I, et al. A systemic review of bisphosphonate osteonecrosis (BON) in cancer. Support Care Cancer 2010;18(8):1099–106.
23. Lee KC, Lee SJ. Clinical features and treatments of odontogenic sinusitis. Yonsei Med J 2010;51(6):932–7.
24. Fox PC, Ship JA. Salivary gland diseases. In: Greenburg MS, Glick M, Ship JA, editors. Burket's oral medicine. 11th edition. Hamilton (Canada): BC Decker; 2008. p. 191–222.

Disorders of the Masticatory Muscles

Scott S. De Rossi, DMD[a,b,c,*], Ilanit Stern, DMD[a],
Thomas P. Sollecito, DMD[d]

KEYWORDS

- Masticatory muscles • Persistent orofacial muscle pain • Myalgia • Myofascial pain
- Temporomandibular joint disorder • Fibromyalgia

KEY POINTS

- It is clear that there are several types of disorders of the masticatory muscles, each of which may have a complex etiology, clinical course, and response to therapy.
- Masticatory muscle disorders include both regional and centrally mediated problems. Host susceptibility plays a role at several stages of these disorders, including pain modulation and response to therapy.
- Disorders of the masticatory muscles must be accurately identified and differentiated from primary temporomandibular joint disorders such as those involving pain from osteoarthritis, disc displacement, or jaw dysfunction.

INTRODUCTION

Muscle disorders involving the masticatory muscles have been considered analogous to skeletal muscle disorders throughout the body.[1,2] However, emerging research has shed new light on the varied etiology, clinical presentation, diagnosis, and treatment of myofascial pain and masticatory muscle disorders.[3–6] This article reviews the etiology and classification of regional masticatory muscle disorders, the clinical examination of the patient, and evidence-based treatment recommendations.

Mechanisms behind masticatory muscle pain include overuse of a normally perfused muscle or ischemia of a normally working muscle, sympathetic reflexes that produce changes in vascular supply and muscle tone, and changes in psychological and emotional states.[7] Neurons mediating pain from skeletal muscle are subject to

[a] Department of Oral health and Diagnostic Sciences, College of Dental Medicine, Georgia Regents University, 1120 15th Street, Augusta, GA 30912, USA; [b] Department of Otolaryngology/ Head & Neck Surgery, Medical College of Georgia, Georgia Regents University, 1120 15th Street, Augusta, GA 30912, USA; [c] Department of Dermatology, Medical College of Georgia, Georgia Regents University, 1120 15th Street, Augusta, GA 30912, USA; [d] Department of Oral Medicine, University of Pennsylvania School of Dental Medicine, 240 South 40th Street, Philadelphia, PA 19104-6030, USA
* Corresponding author. Department of Oral health and Diagnostic Sciences, College of Dental Medicine, Georgia Regents University, 1120 15th Street, Augusta, GA 30912, USA.
E-mail address: sderossi@gru.edu

Dent Clin N Am 57 (2013) 449–464
http://dx.doi.org/10.1016/j.cden.2013.04.007
0011-8532/13/$ – see front matter © 2013 Published by Elsevier Inc.

strong modulatory influences. Bradykinin, serotonin, substance P, prostaglandins, and neuropeptides sensitize nociceptors and can easily sensitize nociceptive endings. Painful conditions of muscle often result in increased sensitivity of peripheral nociceptors and hyperexcitability in the central nervous system with hyperalgesia.[8]

Muscle disorders can be divided into regional disorders, such as myalgia associated with temporomandibular joint (TMJ) disorder, and systemic disorders, such as pain associated with fibromyalgia.[2] The paucity of data on the etiology and pathophysiology of muscle pain limits the ability to clearly delineate all groups of muscle disorders. Frequently the clinician must rely on clinical judgment to establish a diagnosis. It is clear that well-designed controlled trials and additional research is necessary for the development of validated diagnostic criteria and treatment protocols.[3,9–11]

CLASSIFICATION OF MASTICATORY MUSCLE DISORDERS

Chronic myalgia of the muscle of mastication (MOM) is one aspect of temporomandibular disorders (TMDs).[2,3] Historically, clinicians and researchers have subclassified TMDs into intracapsular disorders and masticatory muscle disorders such as local myalgia, myofascial pain, centrally mediated myalgia, myospasm, myositis, myofibrotic contracture, and masticatory muscle neoplastic disease.[9] Conflicting classification schemes and terminology have led to significant confusion among clinicians, and perhaps inaccurate diagnosis and treatment of patients. In fact, many studies continue to group muscle pain and painful TMJ disorders together under the term TMD, although these entities are pathophysiologically and clinically distinct.[3,12–14] Although the most common feature of most masticatory muscle disorders is pain, mandibular dysfunction such as difficulty chewing and mandibular dysfunction may also occur. The clinician needs to differentiate masticatory muscle disorders from the primary TMDs such as those that involve pain associated with osteoarthritis, disc displacement, or jaw dysfunction (**Table 1**).

The clinical features of masticatory muscle disorders are as follows.

Features of Local Myalgia
- Sore MOM with pain in cheeks and temples on chewing, wide opening, and often on waking (eg, nocturnal bruxism)
- Bilateral
- Described as stiff, sore, aching, spasm, tightness, or cramping
- Sensation of muscle stiffness, weakness, fatigue
- Possible reduced mandibular range of motion
- Differential diagnosis: myositis, myofascial pain, neoplasm, fibromyalgia

Features of Myofascial Pain
- Regional dull, aching muscle pain
- Trigger points present and pain referral on palpation with/without autonomic symptoms
- Referred pain often felt as headache
- Trigger points can be inactivated with local anesthetic injection
- Sensation of muscle stiffness and/or malocclusion not verified clinically
- Otologic symptoms including tinnitus, vertigo, and pain
- Headache or toothache
- Decreased range of motion
- Hyperalgesia in region of referred pain
- Differential diagnosis: arthralgia, myositis, local myalgia, neoplasia, fibromyalgia

Table 1
Diagnostic criteria for masticatory muscle disorders

Disorder	Etiology	Diagnostic Criteria
Centrally mediated chronic muscle pain	Chronic generalized muscle pain associated with a comorbid disease	History of prolonged and continuous muscle pain Regional dull, aching pain at rest Pain aggravated by function of affected muscles Pain aggravated by palpation
Myalgia (local)	Acute muscle pain Protective muscle splinting Postexercise soreness Muscle fatigue Pain from ischemia	Regional dull, aching pain during function No or minimal pain at rest Local muscle tenderness on palpation Absence of trigger points and pain referral
Myofascial pain	Chronic regional muscle pain	Regional dull, aching pain at rest Pain aggravated by function of affected muscles Provocation of trigger points alters pain complaint and reveals referral pattern >50% reduction of pain with vapocoolant spray or local anesthetic injection to trigger point followed by stretch
Myofibrotic contracture	Painless shortening of muscles	Limited range of motion Firmness on passive stretch (hard stop) Little or no pain unless involved muscle is forced to lengthen
Myositis	Inflammation secondary to direct trauma or infection	Continuous pain localized in muscle area following injury or infection Diffuse tenderness over entire muscle Pain aggravated by function of affected muscles Moderate to severe decreased range of motion due to pain and swelling
Neoplasia	Benign or malignant	May or may not be painful Anatomic and structural changes Imaging and biopsy needed
Myospasm	Acute involuntary and continuous muscle contraction	Acute onset of pain at rest and during function Markedly decreased range of motion due to continuous involuntary muscle contraction Pain aggravated by function of affected muscles Increased electromyographic activity higher than at rest Sensation of muscle tightness, cramping, or stiffness

Data from de Leeuw R. Orofacial pain: guidelines for assessment, classification, and management. The American Academy of Orofacial Pain. 4th edition. Chicago: Quintessence Publishing Co, Inc; 2008.

Features of Centrally Mediated Myalgia
- Trigger points and pain referral on palpation
- Sensation of muscle stiffness, weakness, and/or fatigue
- Sensation of malocclusion not verified clinically
- Otologic symptoms including tinnitus, vertigo, and pain
- Decreased range of motion
- Hyperalgesia
- No response to treatment directed at painful muscle tissue
- Differential diagnosis: arthralgia, myositis, myofascial pain, local myalgia, neoplasm, fibromyalgia

Features of Myospasm
- Sudden and involuntary muscle contraction
- Acute malocclusion (dependent on muscles involved)
- Decreased range of motion and pain on function and at rest
- Relatively rare disorder in orofacial pain population
- Differential diagnosis: myositis, local myalgia, neoplasm

Features of Myositis
- History of trauma to muscle or source of infection
- Often continuous pain affecting entire affected muscle
- Pain aggravated by function
- Severe limited range of motion

Features of Myofibrotic Contracture
- Not usually painful
- Often follows long period of limited range of motion or disuse (eg, intermaxillary fixation)
- History of infection or trauma is common
- Differential diagnosis: TMJ ankylosis, coronoid hypertrophy

Features of Masticatory Muscle Neoplasia
- Pain may or may not be present
- Anatomic and structural changes: tumors may be in muscles or masticatory spaces
- Swelling, trismus, paresthesias, and pain referred to teeth
- Positive findings on imaging or biopsy

Some clinicians have stressed classifying myogenic disorders based on an anatomic system allowing for a simpler diagnostic process, because evaluation of the patient involves careful palpation of the masticatory muscles and joints.[13,15,16] The clinician needs to determine the etiology and pathophysiology that occur with the various masticatory muscle disorders, such as disorders caused by trauma. A thorough history and clinical examination, an understanding of pain neuroanatomy and neurophysiology, and an in-depth knowledge of research on muscle pain are important.[16–18] Various causes of myogenous pain are summarized in **Table 2**.

Recently a new term, persistent orofacial muscle pain (POMP), has been introduced, to more accurately reflect the interplay between peripheral nociceptive sources in muscles, faulty central nervous system components, and decreased coping

Table 2
Etiology of myogenous pain

Etiology	Criteria
Focal myalgia from direct trauma	History of trauma preceding pain onset Subjective pain in muscles with function Pain reproduced on palpation
Primary myalgia due to parafunction	No history of trauma Subjective pain in muscle with function Pain reproduced on palpation No trigger points
Secondary myalgia due to active local pathology or recent medications	History of recent joint, oral soft tissue, or pulpal disease or medication (eg, serotonin-selective reuptake inhibitors) that coincides with muscle pain Subjective pain in muscle with function Pain reproduced on palpation
Myofascial pain	No history of recent trauma Subjective pain in muscles with function Pain reproduced on palpation Trigger points and pain referral
Diffuse chronic muscle pain and fibromyalgia	Subjective pain in multiple sites aggravated by function Widespread pain involving more than 3 body quadrants >3 mo duration Strong pain on palpation in 11 of 18 body sites

Data from Clark GT, Minakuchi H. Oral appliances. In: Laskin DM, Greene CS, Hylander WL, editors. Temporomandibular disorders: an evidence-based approach to diagnosis and treatment. Chicago: Quintessence; 2006. p. 377–90.

ability.[3] POMP likely shares mechanisms with tension-type headache, regional myofascial pain, and fibromyalgia, and has genetically influenced traits that determine pain modulation and pharmacogenomics interacting with psychological traits to affect disease onset, clinical progression, and pain experience.[3,4] To date, these factors cannot be identified in the individual patient sufficiently enough to tailor focused, mechanism-based treatment. POMP is consistent with the condition often referred to as centrally mediated myalgia and, as such, treatment needs to be redirected from local and regional therapies to systemic and central ones.

CLINICAL EXAMINATION OF THE PATIENT

The most effective approach for the diagnosis masticatory muscle pain involves careful review of the chief complaint, the history of the present illness (**Table 3**), the dental, medical, and psychosocial behavioral histories (**Box 1**), and a comprehensive evaluation of the head and neck including a cranial nerve assessment (**Table 4**).[2] In addition, imaging modalities may be important in ruling out other conditions. No one physical finding can be relied on to establish a diagnosis; rather, a pattern of abnormalities may suggest the source of the problem and diagnosis.[11] However, masticatory muscle tenderness on palpation is the most consistent examination feature present in TMDs.[19–24] In fact, the clinical features that distinguish patients from non-TMD or masticatory muscle pain most consistently reported in the literature are: restricted passive mouth opening without pain; masticatory muscle tenderness on palpation; limited maximal mouth opening; and an uncorrected deviation on maximum mouth opening and tenderness on muscle or joint palpation.[2,19–24]

Table 3
History of the present illness: pain characteristics

Quality	Common patient descriptors: dull, sharp, tight, aching, tired, etc
Location	Unilateral vs bilateral Pain confined to a single muscle or referred to a distant area
Intensity	On a scale of 1–10 Mild, moderate, or severe
Onset, duration, pattern	How long has the pain been present? What if anything caused the pain? (eg, trauma) What has been the course of pain since its onset? (eg, episodic, constant, fluctuating)
Modifiers	What exacerbates or diminishes the pain? Does anything you do or use help or worsen pain?
Chronicity	How long has the pain been present?
Comorbid symptoms and signs	Are there any other conditions or symptoms associated with pain? (eg, depression, acute anxiety, nausea/vomiting, tearing, visual changes, dizziness, numbness/tingling, weakness, generalized pain)

Box 1
Questions regarding oral behavior and parafunction

DO YOU:

Clench or grind your teeth when asleep?

Sleep in a position that puts pressure on your jaw? (eg, side, stomach)

Clench or press teeth together while awake?

Touch or hold teeth together while eating?

Hold, tighten, or tense muscles without clenching or touching teeth together?

Hold out or jut jaw forward or to side?

Press tongue between teeth?

Bite, chew, or play with tongue, cheeks, or lips?

Hold jaw in rigid or tense position to brace or protect jaw?

Bite or hold objects between teeth (eg, pens, pipe, hair, fingernails, and so forth)?

Use chewing gum?

Play musical instruments that involve mouth or jaw?

Lean with hand on jaw or chin?

Chew food on one side only?

Eat between meals (food requiring lots of chewing)?

Talk at length?

Sing?

Yawn excessively?

Hold telephone between head and shoulder?

Data from Ohrbach R, Markiewicz M, McCall WD Jr. Oral Behaviors Checklist: performance validity of targeted behaviors [abstract]. J Dent Res 2004;83:(Spec Issue A):T27–45.

Table 4
Physical examination directed toward mandibular dysfunction

Examination	Observations
Inspection	Facial asymmetry, swelling, and masseter and temporal muscle hypertrophy Opening pattern (corrected and uncorrected deviations, uncoordinated movements, limitations)
Assessment of range of mandibular movement	Maximum opening with comfort, with pain, and with clinician assistance Maximum lateral and protrusive movements
Palpation examination	Masticatory muscles Temporomandibular joints Neck muscles and accessory muscles of the jaw Parotid and submandibular areas Lymph nodes
Provocation tests	Static pain test (mandibular resistance against pressure) Pain in the joints or muscles with tooth clenching Reproduction of symptoms with chewing (wax, sugarless gum)
Intraoral examination	Signs of parafunction (cheek or lip biting, accentuated linea alba, scalloped tongue borders, occlusal wear, tooth mobility, generalized sensitivity to percussion, thermal testing, multiple fractures of enamel, restorations)

Data from Refs.[2,19–24,27]

Objective determination of the presence or absence of parafunctional jaw behavior is challenging.[25] Although the presence of these behaviors may not have proven diagnostic validity, their assessment remains important because it provides potential causative or perpetual factors and/or effects on the masticatory system.[26] An oral behavior checklist is a useful instrument for determining the presence or awareness of parafunctional behaviors.[27]

Interincisor separation (plus or minus the incisor overlap in centric occlusion) provides the measure of mandibular movement. Maximum interincisal opening (MIO) should be measured using a ruler without pain, as wide as possible with pain, and after opening with clinician assistance. Mouth opening with assistance is accomplished by applying mild to moderate pressure against the upper and lower incisors with the thumb and index finger. Passive stretching often allows the clinician to assess and differentiate the limitation of opening caused by a muscle or joint problem by comparing assisted opening with active opening. This action provides the examiner with the quality of resistance at the end of the movement. Often, muscle restrictions are associated with a soft end-feel and result in an increase of more than 5 mm above the active opening (wide opening with pain), whereas joint disorders such as acute nonreducing disc displacements have a hard end-feel and characteristically limit assisted opening to less than 5 mm (normal MIO is ~40 mm; range 35–55 mm). Measurements of lateral movement are made with the teeth slightly separated, measuring the displacement of the lower midline from the maxillary midline, and adding or subtracting the lower-midline displacement at the start of movement. Protrusive movement is measured by adding the horizontal distance between the upper and lower central incisors and adding the distance the lower incisors travel beyond the upper incisors; normal lateral and protrusive movements are approximately 7 mm.

The primary finding related to masticatory muscle palpation is pain; however, the methods for palpation are not standardized in clinical practice.[28] The amount of pressure to apply and the exact sites that are most likely associated with TMD are unknown. Some clinicians have recommended attempting to establish a baseline (to serve as a general guide or reference) by squeezing a muscle between the index finger and thumb or by applying pressure in the center of the forehead or thumbnail to gauge what pressure becomes uncomfortable.[9] The Research Diagnostic Criteria for Temporomandibular Disorders (RDC/TMD) guidelines recommend 1 lb (0.45 kg) of pressure for the joint and 2 lb (0.9 kg) of pressure for the muscles. Palpation should be accompanied by: asking the patient about the presence of pain at the palpation site; whether palpation produces pain spread or referral to a distant site; and whether palpation reproduces the pain the patient has been experiencing.[9,29] Reproducing the site and the character of the pain during the examination procedure helps identify the potential source of the pain. The distant origin of referred pain can also be identified by palpation.[29]

Palpation of the muscles for pain should be done with the muscles in a resting state.[29] There are no standardized methods of assessing the severity of palpable pain, and the patient should be asked to rate the severity by using a scale (eg, a numeric scale from 1 to 10, a visual analog scale, or a ranking such as none, mild, moderate, or severe). The RDC/TMD recommends using the categories of pressure only, mild pain, moderate pain, and severe pain.[9] These ratings may also be useful in assessing treatment progress in addition to asking patients what percentage of improvement they may feel. The lateral pterygoid is in a position that does not allow access for adequate palpation examination, even though there are examination protocols and descriptions for palpating this muscle.

Patients with TMDs often have musculoskeletal problems in other regions (neck, back, and so forth).[30] The upper cervical somatosensory nerves send branches that synapse in the spinal trigeminal nucleus, which is one proposed mechanism to explain referral of pain from the neck to the orofacial region and masticatory muscles.[31–33] The sternocleidomastoid and trapezius muscles are often part of cervical muscle disorders, and may refer pain to the face and head. Other cervical muscle groups to include in the palpation examination include the paravertebral (scalene) and suboccipital muscles.

Injections of anesthetics into the TMJ or selected masticatory muscles may help confirm a diagnosis. Elimination of or a significant decrease in pain and improved jaw motion should be considered a positive test result. Diagnostic injections may also be helpful in differentiating pain arising from joints or muscle.[2,29] In situations where a joint procedure is being considered, local anesthetic injection of the joint may confirm the joint as the source of pain. Injecting trigger points or tender areas of muscle should eliminate pain from the site and should also eliminate referred pain associated with the injected trigger point. Interpretation of injections in the context of all the diagnostic information is vital, because a positive result does not ensure a specific diagnosis. Recently, the use of botulinum toxin (Botox) has been advocated for trigger-point injections and for the management of tension-type headache.[3,4,6,29] In several case-control studies and randomized trials, descriptive analysis showed that improvements in both objective (range of mandibular movements) and subjective (pain at rest; pain during chewing) clinical outcome variables were higher in Botox-treated groups than in the placebo-treated subjects. Patients treated with Botox had a higher subjective improvement in their perception of treatment efficacy than placebo-treated subjects.[2,6,29]

TREATMENT OF MASTICATORY MUSCLE DISORDERS

It is important for the clinician treating patients with TMDs to distinguish clinically significant disorders that require therapy from incidental findings in a patient with facial pain attributable to other causes.[2] TMJ abnormalities are often discovered on routine examination, and may not require treatment such as with asymptomatic clicking of the TMJ. The need for treatment is largely based on the level of pain and dysfunction as well as the progression of symptoms. With respect to disorders of MOM, the principles of treatment are based on a generally favorable prognosis and an appreciation of the lack of clinically controlled trials indicating the superiority, predictability, and safety of treatments presently available. The literature suggests that many treatments have some beneficial effect, although this effect may be nonspecific and not directly related to the particular treatment.[1–3,9]

According to the American Association of Dental Research, it is strongly recommended that, unless there are specific and justifiable indications to the contrary, treatment of TMD patients, including those with disorders of MOM, initially should be based on the use of conservative, reversible, and evidence-based therapeutic modalities.[34] Studies of the natural history of many TMDs suggest that they tend to improve or resolve over time.[12,14,15,19,21,35] Although no specific therapies have been proved to be uniformly effective, many of the conservative modalities have proved to be at least as effective as most forms of invasive treatment in providing symptomatic relief. Because such modalities do not produce irreversible changes, they present much less risk of producing harm. Professional treatment should be augmented with a home-care program whereby patients are taught about their disorder and how to manage their symptoms.[34,36]

Treatments that are relatively accessible, not prohibitive owing to expense, safe, and reversible should be given priority, for example: education; self-care; physical therapy; intraoral appliance therapy; and short-term pharmacotherapy, behavioral therapy, and relaxation techniques (**Table 5**). There is evidence to suggest that multimodal therapy and combining treatments produces a better outcome.[5,37] Occlusal therapy continues to be recommended by some clinicians as an initial treatment or as a requirement to prevent recurrent symptoms. However, research does not support occlusal abnormalities as a significant etiologic factor in TMD including masticatory muscle disorders.[2,38–41]

Avoidance therapy and cognitive awareness plays a vital role in patient care but has little scientific evidence to support its use.[2,17,24,25] Generally speaking, common sense dictates that if something hurts, it should be avoided. Four behaviors should be avoided in the patient with masticatory muscle pain:

1. Avoidance of clenching by reproducing a rest position where the patient's lips are closed but teeth are slightly separated
2. Avoidance of poor head and neck posture
3. Avoidance of testing the jaw or jaw joint clicking
4. Avoidance of other habits such as nail biting, lip biting, gum chewing, and so forth (**Box 2**).

Many patients report benefit from heat or ice packs applied to painful MOM. The local application of heat can increase circulation and relax muscles, whereas ice may serve as an anesthetic for painful muscles. In addition, stretch therapy must be part of a self-care program. Stretches should be done multiple times daily to maximize effectiveness. The most effective stretching exercise is passive stretching, summarized in **Box 3**.

Table 5 Initial treatment of masticatory muscle disorders	
Treatment Component	**Description**
Education	Explanation of the diagnosis and treatment Reassurance about the generally good prognosis for recovery and natural course Explanation of patient's and doctor's roles in therapy Information to enable patient to perform self-care
Self-care	Eliminate oral habits (eg, tooth clenching, chewing gum) Provide information on jaw care associated with daily activities
Physical therapy	Education regarding biomechanics of jaw, neck, and head posture Passive modalities (heat and cold therapy, ultrasound, laser, TENS) Range of motion exercises (active and passive) Posture therapy Passive stretching, general exercise and conditioning program
Intraoral appliance therapy	Cover all the teeth on the arch the appliance is seated on Adjust to achieve simultaneous contact against opposing teeth Adjust to a stable comfortable mandibular posture Avoid changing mandibular position Avoid long-term continuous use
Pharmacotherapy	NSAIDs, acetaminophen, muscle relaxants, antianxiety agents, tricyclic antidepressants
Behavioral/relaxation techniques	Relaxation therapy Hypnosis Biofeedback Cognitive-behavioral therapy

Abbreviations: NSAIDs, nonsteroidal anti-inflammatory drugs; TENS, transcutaneous electrical nerve stimulation.
Data from Refs.[2,17,40,41]

Physiotherapy helps to relieve musculoskeletal pain and restore normal function by altering sensory input; reducing inflammation; decreasing, coordinating, and strengthening muscle activity; and promoting the rehabilitation of tissues.[14] A licensed professional therapist is recommended for treatment. Despite the absence of well-controlled clinical trials, physiotherapy is a well-recognized effective and conservative therapy for many disorders of the MOM.

Physical Therapy Techniques
- Posture training
- Exercises
- Mobilization

Physical Agents and Modalities
- Electrotherapy and transcutaneous electrical nerve stimulations (TENS)
- Ultrasound
- Iontophoresis
- Vapocoolant spray
- Trigger-point injections with local anesthetic or Botox
- Acupuncture
- Laser treatment

Box 2
Patient's instructions for self-care

- Be aware of habits or patterns of jaw use.
  - Avoid tooth contact except during chewing and swallowing.
  - Notice any contact the teeth make.
  - Notice any clenching, grinding, gritting, or tapping of teeth, or any tensing or rigid holding of the jaw muscles.
  - Check for tooth clenching while driving, studying, doing computer work, reading, or engaging in athletic activities; when at work or in social situations; and when experiencing overwork, fatigue, or stress.
  - Position the jaw to avoid tooth contacts.
  - Place the tip of the tongue behind the top teeth and keep the teeth slightly apart; maintain this position when the jaw is not being used for functions such as speaking and chewing.
- Modify your diet.
  - Choose softer foods and only those foods that can be chewed without pain.
  - Cut foods into smaller pieces; avoid foods that require wide mouth opening and biting off with the front teeth, or foods that are chewy and sticky and that require excessive mouth movements.
  - Do not chew gum.
- Do not test the jaw.
- Do not open the mouth wide or move the jaw around excessively to assess pain or motion.
- Avoid habitually maneuvering the jaw into positions to assess its comfort or range.
- Avoid habitually clicking the jaw if a click is present.
- Avoid certain postures.
  - Do not lean on or cup the chin when performing desk work or at the dining table.
  - Do not sleep on the stomach or in postures that place stress on the jaw.
- Avoid elective dental treatment while symptoms of pain and limited opening are present.
- During yawning, support the jaw by providing mild pressure underneath the chin with the thumb and index finger or with the back of the hand.
- Apply moist hot compresses to the sides of the face and to the temple areas for 10 to 20 minutes twice daily.

SPLINT THERAPY

Splints, orthotics, orthopedic appliances, bite guards, nightguards, or bruxing guards are used in TMD treatment, and often for disorders of masticatory muscles.[2] Their use is considered to be a reversible part of initial therapy. Several studies on splint therapy have demonstrated a treatment effect, although researchers disagree as to the reason for the effect.[5,14,15] In a review of the literature on splint therapy, Clark and colleagues[17,24] found that patients reported a 70% to 90% improvement with splint therapy. A recent review of the research on splint therapy suggests that using a splint as part of therapy for masticatory myalgia, arthralgia, or both may be supported by the literature in case-control studies.[40] Conversely, there is insufficient evidence on review of published randomized controlled trials to support the use of stabilization splint

Box 3
Patient's exercise instructions

Certain exercises can help you relieve the pain that comes from tired, cramped muscles. They can also help if you have difficulty opening your mouth. The exercises described work by helping you relax tense muscles and are referred to as "passive stretching." The more often you do these exercises, the more you'll relax the muscles that are painfully tense.

Do these exercises 2 times daily:

1. Ice down both sides of the face for 5 to 10 minutes before beginning (ice cubes in sandwich bags or packs of frozen vegetables work well for this).

2. Place thumb of one hand on the edge of the upper front teeth and the index and middle fingers of the other hand on the edge of the lower front teeth, with the thumb under the chin.

3. The starting position for the stretches is with the thumb of the one hand and index finger of the other hand just touching.

4. Gently pull open the lower jaw, using the hand only, until you feel a passive stretch, not pain, hold for 10 seconds, then allow the lower jaw to close until the thumb and index finger are once again contacting; it is crucial that when doing these exercises not to use the jaw muscles to open and close, but rather manual manipulation only (the fingers do all the work!).

5. Repeat the above stretching action 10 times, performing 2 to 3 sets per day, 1 in the morning and 1 or 2 in the evening.

6. When finished with the exercises, one can place moist heat to both sides of the face for 5 to 10 minutes (heating a wet washcloth in the microwave for about 1 minute works well for this).

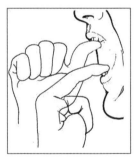

Demonstration of a passive stretch using the fingers.

therapy over other active interventions in the treatment of myofascial pain. Splints appear to be better than no treatment, but only as effective as other active interventions for myofascial pain.[40–43] A systematic review and meta-analysis by Ebrahim and colleagues[37] reviewed 11 eligible studies of 1567 patients, and demonstrated promising results for pain reduction, very low evidence for an effect on quality of life, and significant research bias (**Box 4**).

PHARMACOLOGIC THERAPY

Both clinical and controlled experimental studies suggest that medications may promote patient comfort and rehabilitation when used as part of comprehensive

Box 4
Splint therapy
• The appliance most commonly used is described as a stabilization appliance or muscle relaxation splint
• Designed to cover a full arch and adjusted to avoid altering jaw position or placing orthodontic forces on the teeth ○ Should be adjusted to provide bilateral, even contact with the opposing teeth on closure and in a comfortable mandibular posture ○ Should be reexamined periodically and readjusted as necessary to accommodate changes in mandibular posture or muscle function that may affect the opposing tooth contacts on the appliance
• At the beginning of appliance therapy, a combination of appliance use during sleep and for periods during waking hours is appropriate ○ Factors such as tooth clenching when driving or exercising, or pain symptoms that tend to increase as the day progresses, may be better managed by increasing splint use during these times
• To avoid the possibility of occlusal change, no appliance should not be worn continuously (ie, 24 hours per day) over prolonged periods
• Full-coverage appliance therapy during sleep is a common practice to reduce the effects of bruxism and is not usually associated with occlusal change

treatment. Although there is a tendency for clinicians to rely on "favorite" agents, no single medication has proved to be effective for the entire spectrum of TMDs.[2–4,17,24] With respect to pain associated with disorders of the MOM, analgesics, nonsteroidal anti-inflammatory agents, corticosteroids, benzodiazepines, muscle relaxants, and low-dose antidepressants have shown efficacy. Many of the medications used for fibromyalgia can be used for patients with masticatory muscle disorders (**Table 6**).[30] These agents are versatile and effective at treating the multiple symptoms associated with chronic muscle pain. The medications used for myofascial pain and masticatory muscle disorders are discussed in greater detail elsewhere in this issue by Nasri-Heir and colleagues.

Table 6
Medications used for fibromyalgia that may be beneficial for masticatory muscle pain

Medication Class	Effect
Tricyclic antidepressants (TCAs)	Moderately helpful for pain More side effects (xerostomia, fatigue)
Serotonin-selective reuptake inhibitors	Fewer side effects than TCAs More effective for anxiety/depression than for pain
Muscle relaxants	Moderately helpful for local muscle pain More side effects (xerostomia, sedation)
Serotonin-norepinephrine reuptake inhibitors	Moderately helpful for fibromyalgia-related pain
Low-potency opioids	Moderately helpful for fibromyalgia-related pain
NSAIDs	Helpful for acute inflammatory pain but not chronic muscle pain or fibromyalgia-related pain

SUMMARY

It is clear that there are several types of disorders of the masticatory muscles, each of which may have a complex etiology, clinical course, and response to therapy. Masticatory muscle disorders include both regional and centrally mediated problems. Host susceptibility plays a role at several stages of these disorders, including pain modulation and response to therapy. Disorders of the masticatory muscles must be accurately identified and differentiated from primary TMJ disorders such as those involving pain from osteoarthritis, disc displacement, or jaw dysfunction.[44]

REFERENCES

1. Waltimo A, Kemppainen P, Kononen M. Maximal contraction force and endurance of human jaw closing muscles in isometric clenching. Scand J Dent Res 1993; 101:416–21.
2. Scrivani SJ, Keith DA, Kaban LB. Temporomandibular disorders. N Engl J Med 2008;359:2693–705.
3. Benoliel R, Svensson P, Heir GM, et al. Persistent orofacial muscle pain. Oral Dis 2011;17(Suppl 1):23–41.
4. Benoliel R, Sharav Y. Chronic orofacial pain. Curr Pain Headache Rep 2010;14: 33–40.
5. Galdon MJ, Dura E, Andreu Y, et al. Multidimensional approach to the differences between muscular and articular temporomandibular patients: coping, distress, and pain characteristics. Oral Surg Oral Med Oral Pathol 2006;102:40–6.
6. Myburgh C, Larsen AH, Hartvifgsen J. A systematic, critical review of manual palpation for identifying myofascial trigger points: evidence and clinical significance. Arch Phys Med Rehabil 2008;89:1169–76.
7. Nijs J, Daenen L, Cras P, et al. Nociception affects motor output: a review on sensory-motor interaction with focus on clinical implications. Clin J Pain 2012; 28(2):175–81.
8. Staud R. Is it all central sensitization? Role of peripheral tissue nociception in chronic musculoskeletal pain. Curr Rheumatol Rep 2010;12(6):448–54.
9. Dworkin SF, LeResche L. Research Diagnostic Criteria for temporomandibular disorders: review, criteria, examinations and specifications, critique. J Craniomandib Disord 1992;6:302–55.
10. Look JO, John MT, Tai F, et al. The research diagnostic criteria for temporomandibular disorders II: reliability of Axis I diagnoses and selected clinical measures. J Orofac Pain 2010;24:25–34.
11. Mohl ND. The anecdotal tradition and the need for evidence-based care for temporomandibular disorders. J Orofac Pain 1999;13:227–31.
12. Dworkin S, Huggins K, LeResche L, et al. Epidemiology of signs and symptoms in temporomandibular disorders: clinical signs in cases and controls. J Am Dent Assoc 1990;120:273–81.
13. Anderson GC, Gonzalez YM, Ohrbach R, et al. The research diagnostic criteria for temporomandibular disorders. VI: future directions. J Orofac Pain 2010;24: 19–88.
14. de Leeuw R. Orofacial pain: guidelines for assessment, classification, and management. The American Academy of Orofacial Pain. 4th edition. Chicago: Quintessence Publishing Co., Inc; 2008.
15. Lobbezo F, Drangsholt M, Peck C, et al. Topical review: new insights into the pathology and diagnosis of the temporomandibular joint. J Orofac Pain 2004;18: 181–91.

16. Sessle BJ. The neural basis of temporomandibular joint and masticatory muscle pain. J Orofac Pain 1999;13:238–45.
17. Clark GT, Minakuchi H. Oral appliances. In: Laskin DM, Greene CS, Hylander WL, editors. Temporomandibular disorders: an evidence-based approach to diagnosis and treatment. Chicago: Quintessence; 2006. p. 377–90.
18. Lund JP. Muscular pain and dysfunction. In: Laskin DM, Greene CS, Hylander WL, editors. Temporomandibular disorders: an evidence-based approach to diagnosis and treatment. Chicago: Quintessence; 2006. p. 99.
19. Schiffman E, Fricton JR, Haley D, et al. The prevalence and treatment needs of subjects with temporomandibular disorders. J Am Dent Assoc 1989;120:295–301.
20. Lipton JA, Ship JA, Larach-Robinson D. Estimated prevalence and distributions of orofacial pain in the United States. J Am Dent Assoc 1993;124:115–21.
21. Kurita K, Westesson PL, Yuasa H, et al. Natural course of untreated symptomatic temporomandibular joint disc displacement without reduction. J Dent Res 1998; 77:361–5.
22. Milam SB. TMJ osteoarthritis. In: Laskin DM, Greene CS, Hylander WL, editors. Temporomandibular disorders: an evidence-based approach to diagnosis and treatment. Chicago: Quintessence; 2006. p. 105–23.
23. Rammelsberg P, Leresche L, Dworkin S, et al. Longitudinal outcome of temporomandibular disorders: a 5-year epidemiologic study of muscle disorders defined by Research Diagnostic Criteria for Temporomandibular Disorders. J Orofac Pain 2003;17:9–20.
24. Clark GT, Seligman DA, Solberg WK, et al. Guidelines for the examination and diagnosis of temporomandibular disorders. J Craniomandib Disord 1989;3:7–14.
25. Dworkin SF. Psychological and psychosocial assessment. In: Laskin DM, Greene CS, Hylander WL, editors. Temporomandibular disorders: an evidence-based approach to diagnosis and treatment. Chicago: Quintessence; 2006. p. 203–17.
26. Fricton J, Kroening R, Hathaway K. TMJ and craniofacial pain: diagnosis and management. St Louis (MO): Ishiyaku Euroamerica; 1988.
27. Ohrbach R, Markiewicz M, McCall WD Jr. Oral Behaviors Checklist: performance validity of targeted behaviors [abstract]. J Dent Res 2004;83(Spec Issue A): T27–45.
28. National Institutes of Health Technology Assessment Conference on Management of Temporomandibular Disorders. Oral Surg Oral Med Oral Pathol Oral Radiol Endod 1997;83:49–183.
29. Simons DG. Neurophysiologic basis of pain caused by trigger points. APS J 1994;3:17–9.
30. Clauw DJ. Fibromyalgia: an overview. Am J Med 2009;122:S3–13.
31. Diatchenko L, Slade GD, Nackley AG, et al. Genetic basis for individual variations in pain perception and the development of a chronic pain condition. Hum Mol Genet 2005;14:135–43.
32. Fillingim RD. Sex differences in analgesic responses: evidence from experimental pain models. Eur J Anaesthesiol Suppl 2002;26:16–24.
33. Raphael KG, Marbach JJ, Gallagher RM. Somatosensory amplification and affective inhibition are elevated in myofascial face pain. Pain Med 2000;1:247–53.
34. Greene CS. Managing the care of patients with temporomandibular disorders: a new guideline for care. J Am Dent Assoc 2010;141(9):1086–8.
35. Wanman A. Longitudinal course of symptoms of craniomandibular disorders in men and women. A 10-year follow-up study of an epidemiologic sample. Acta Odontol Scand 1996;54:337–42.

36. Glaros AG, Burton E. Parafunctional clenching, pain, and effort in temporomandibular disorders. J Behav Med 2004;27:91–100.
37. Ebrahim S, Montoya L, Busse JW, et al. The effectiveness of splint therapy in patients with temporomandibular disorders. J Am Dent Assoc 2012;143:847–57.
38. Henrikson T, Nilner M. Temporomandibular disorders, occlusion and orthodontic treatment. J Orthod 2003;30:129–37.
39. Poggio CE, Schmitz JH, Worthington HV, et al. Interventions for myogenous temporomandibular disorder (TMD) patients. Cochrane Database Syst Rev 2010;11:CD008828.
40. Kreiner M, Betancor E, Clark GT. Occlusal stabilization appliances. Evidence of their efficacy. J Am Dent Assoc 2001;132:770–7.
41. Fricton J, Look JO, Wright E. Systematic review and meta-analysis of randomized controlled trials evaluating intraoral orthopedic appliances for temporomandibular disorders. J Orofac Pain 2010;24:237–54.
42. Truelove E, Huggins KH, Mancl L, et al. The efficacy of traditional, low-cost and nonsplint therapies for temporomandibular disorders: a randomized clinical trial. J Am Dent Assoc 2006;137:1099–107.
43. Michelotti A, Iodice G, Vollaro S, et al. Evaluation of the short-term effectiveness of education versus an occlusal splint for the treatment of myofascial pain of the jaw muscles. J Am Dent Assoc 2012;143:47–53.
44. Klasser GD, Greene CS. The changing field of temporomandibular disorders: what dentists need to know. J Can Dent Assoc 2009;75(1):49–53.

Epidemiology, Diagnosis, and Treatment of Temporomandibular Disorders

Frederick Liu, DDS, MD*, Andrew Steinkeler, DMD, MD

KEYWORDS

- Temporomandibular disorders • Epidemiology • Diagnosis • Treatment

KEY POINTS

- Temporomandibular disorder (TMD) is a multifactorial disease process caused by muscle hyperfunction or parafunction, traumatic injuries, hormonal influences, and articular changes.
- Symptoms of TMD include decreased mandibular range of motion, muscle and joint pain, joint crepitus, and functional limitation or deviation of the jaw opening.
- Only after failure of noninvasive options should more invasive and nonreversible treatments be initiated.
- Treatment can be divided into noninvasive, minimally invasion, and invasive options.
- Temporomandibular joint replacement is reserved for severely damaged joints with end-stage disease that has failed all other more conservative treatment modalities.

EPIDEMIOLOGY

Temporomandibular disorders (TMD) are a broad group of clinical problems involving the masticatory musculature, the temporomandibular joint, surrounding bony and soft tissue components, and combinations of these problems.[1] Symptoms of TMD include decreased mandibular range of motion, pain in the muscles of mastication, temporomandibular joint (TMJ) pain, associated joint noise with function, generalized myofascial pain, and a functional limitation or deviation of the jaw opening.[1] The prevalence of TMD is thought to be greater than 5% of the population.[2] Lipton and colleagues[3] showed that about 6% to 12% of the population experience clinical symptoms of TMD. Patients with TMD symptoms present over a broad age range; however, there is a peak occurrence between 20 and 40 years of age.[4]

Department of Oral and Maxillofacial Surgery, School of Dental Medicine, University of Pennsylvania, 3400 Spruce Street, Philadelphia, PA 19103, USA
* Corresponding author.
E-mail address: fred.liu@gmail.com

Dent Clin N Am 57 (2013) 465–479
http://dx.doi.org/10.1016/j.cden.2013.04.006
0011-8532/13/$ – see front matter © 2013 Elsevier Inc. All rights reserved.

TMD symptoms are more prevalent in women than men. Contrary to the known increased health risk in postmenopausal women of conditions such as heart disease and stroke, women tend to develop TMD during their premenopausal years.[1] The reasons behind the sexual disequilibrium in TMD prevalence are not entirely clear, but some have suggested a hormonal influence.[5–7] In fact, both animal and human studies have suggested that sex hormones may predispose to TMJ dysfunction and cartilaginous breakdown.[5–7] Elevated levels of estrogen have been found in patients with TMD.[1] However, no definitive link between these hormones and causation of TMD has been established.

TMD is thought to be a multifactorial process secondary to muscle hyperfunction or parafunction, traumatic injuries, hormonal influences, and articular changes within the joint. Various investigators have found correlations between occlusion and TMJ symptoms. Mohlin and Kopp[8] showed an association between occlusal interferences and myofascial pain and dysfunction. They found links between posterior crossbite with muscular discomfort. Patients with deep bites, class II malocclusion, and anterior open bites may also be predisposed to myofascial pain.[9–12]

DIAGNOSIS AND CLASSIFICATION

In general, TMD can be divided into articular and nonarticular disorders. These disorders are synonymous with intracapsular and extracapsular conditions, respectively. Most nonarticular disorders present as myofascial pain focused to the muscles of mastication (**Fig. 1**). In fact, more than 50% of TMD is myofascial pain. Other nonarticular disorders include chronic conditions, such as fibromyalgia, muscle strain, and myopathies. Myofascial pain and dysfunction is theorized to arise from clenching, bruxism, or other parafunctional habits. The result is masticatory musculature strain, spasm, pain, and functional limitation.[2] Emotional stress also predisposes to clenching and bruxism, which contributes to myofascial pain.[13] Symptoms include chronic pain in the masticatory muscles, radiating pain to the ears, neck, and head. Myofascial pain can be treated with combinations of nonsteroidal antiinflammatory medications, occlusal guards, physical therapy, muscle relaxants, and injectable local anesthetic/steroid combinations into the masticatory muscle insertion points.

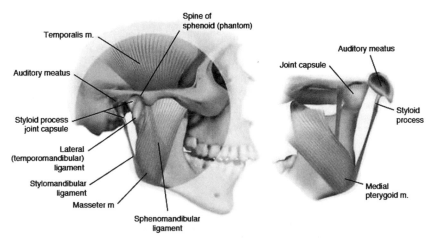

Fig. 1. Musculoskeletal structures of TMJ (lateral and medial views).

Articular disorders (internal derangement) can be divided into inflammatory and noninflammatory arthropathies. Inflammatory articular disorders include rheumatologic processes, such as rheumatoid arthritis (RA), seronegative spondylopathies, such as ankylosing spondylitis, psoriatic arthritis, gout, and infectious arthritis. Noninflammatory articular disk disorders include osteoarthritis, joint damage from prior trauma or surgery, or other cartilage or bone disorders (**Table 1**). Mechanistically, articular disorders occur as a result of an altered balance of anabolic and catabolic cytokines. This cytokine imbalance creates an inflammatory milieu, which leads to oxidative stress, free radicals, and ultimately joint damage.[2]

Internal derangement equates to changes in the disk-condyle relationship.[14] Disk displacements are categorized as disk displacement with reduction or disk displacement without reduction (**Fig. 2**). The fibrocartilage disk is typically displaced anteromedially but rarely may be displaced laterally or posteriorly.[15–17] Anatomically, disk displacement with reduction is interference between the mandibular condyle with the articular disk during jaw opening or closing. This interference may generate clicking, popping, or crepitus in the joint, which can be associated with discomfort. Clicking alone, however, is not diagnostic of articular disk displacement. During disk displacement with reduction, the condyle meets the posterior aspect of the disk, which then reduces to its proper position between the condyle and glenoid fossa.[14,17] Articular disk displacement is associated with TMD. One study found magnetic resonance imaging (MRI) evidence of disk displacement in 84% of symptomatic patients with TMD versus 33% of asymptomatic patients.[18] MRI findings, however, should not solely dictate treatment because disk displacement may occur in asymptomatic patients. Disk displacement without reduction results in a closed lock whereby the condylar movement is physically blocked by the anteriorly displaced disk. Acute closed clock is associated with limited mandibular opening and severe pain.[14,17] Physical examination should include a general assessment of the head and neck, palpation of the masticatory muscles, occlusal analysis, examination of the jaw opening and closing, and palpation of the TMJ. Palpation of the muscles of mastication may elicit mild to severe pain. Masseters are palpated with fingers positioned over the angle of the mandible. The temporalis muscles are palpated along the temple with the jaw relaxed and clenched. The pterygoid muscles are palpated intraorally along the medial aspect of the mandibular ramus between the tonsillar pillars.

Table 1
Articular and nonarticular disorders

Articular Disorders	Nonarticular Disorders
Osteoarthritis	Myofascial pain
Trauma	Acute muscle strain
Infectious arthritis	Muscle spasm
Prior surgery (iatrogenic)	Fibromyalgia
Gout/pseudogout (crystal-arthropathies)	Chronic pain conditions
Rheumatoid arthritis/juvenile RA	Myotonic dystrophy
Psoriatic arthritis	
Ankylosing spondylitis	

Adapted from Ghali GE, Miloro M, Waite PD, et al, editors. Peterson's principles of oral and maxillofacial surgery. 3rd edition. Shelton (CT): People's Medical Publishing House—USA; 2012. ISBN-10: 1-60795-111-8, ISBN-13: 978-1-60795-111-7. STAT!Ref Online Electronic Medical Library. Available at: http://online.statref.com/document.aspx?fxid=100&docid=1212. Accessed January 26, 2013. 1:56:41 PM CST (UTC -06:00).

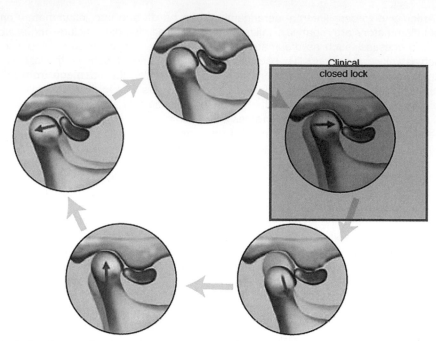

Fig. 2. Motion mechanics seen in temporomandibular joint with anteriorly displaced disc and resultant closed lock.

In general, articular disorders are classified according to the Wilkes' Staging Classification for Internal Derangement of the TMJ (stages I–V). Wilkes' classification is based on clinical, radiologic, and anatomic findings (**Box 1**).[19] For research purposes, a more detailed diagnostic classification is used. This classification is known as the Research Diagnostic Criteria for TMD (RDC/TMD). The RDC/TMD classification system is divided into 3 axes: axis I (muscle disorders), axis 2 (disk disorders), and axis 3 (arthralgias).[20]

Diagnosing TMD requires a focused history and physical examination. Pain and limited range of motion are accepted symptoms of TMJ dysfunction. Radiographic studies can also be used as supplemental diagnostic tools.

Periapical radiographs can be used to rule out dental pathologies as a cause of referred pain. Cone beam computed tomography scans and panoramic radiographs will provide detailed imaging of the joint's bony structures but not the articular disk. MRI is the modality of choice for examining the disk position and morphology (gold standard). MRI may also show degenerative bony changes. MRI findings should not alone dictate treatment strategies. One must combine patients' clinical presentation, signs, and symptoms along with TMJ imaging when developing a treatment plan. On MRI, joint effusions are radiographic signs of inflammation.[21] Inflammation indicates a transition from adaptive to pathologic changes within the joint. The MRI diagnosis of anterior disk displacement uses the most superior aspect of the condyle (12-o'clock position) as a reference point.[21] Anterior disk displacement is defined radiographically when the posterior disk tissue is located anterior to the 12-o'clock condylar position. Disk displacement may occur in asymptomatic patients such that all radiographic findings must be placed in clinical context before beginning TMJ treatments.

Box 1
Wilkes' staging for internal derangement of the TMJ

I. Early stage

   A. Clinical presentation: no pain or decreased range of motion, possible clicking

   B. Radiographic presentation: disk anteriorly positioned, normal bony contours

   C. Anatomic correlation: anterior displacement, normal anatomic form of bone, and disk

II. Early/intermediate stage

   A. Clinical presentation: episodes of pain, opening clicks, intermittent locking

   B. Radiographic presentation: anterior disk displacement, thickened posterior disk, bony contours normal

   C. Anatomic correlation: early disk deformity, anterior displacement, normal bony contours

III. Intermediate stage

   A. Clinical presentation: many painful episodes, intermittent closed locking, multiple functional symptoms, decreased range of motion

   B. Radiographic presentation: anterior disk displacement with disk deformity

   C. Anatomic correlation: marked disk displacement and deformity, normal bony contours

IV. Intermediate/late stage

   A. Clinical presentation: increased pain relative to earlier stages

   B. Radiographic presentation: bony changes, such as flattened eminence, condylar deformity, osteosclerotic changes

   C. Anatomic correlation: adhesions of disk, bony changes, evidence of osteoarthritis, osteophytes, no disk perforations

V. Late stage

   A. Clinical presentation: episodic or continuous pain, crepitus, limited range of motion at all times, constant functional difficulties

   B. Radiographic presentation: disk perforations, gross deformities of bony structures and cartilage, progressive arthritic changes

   C. Anatomic correlation: gross hard and soft tissue changes, perforations, adhesions, subcortical cysts

Adapted from Bronstein S, Merrill B. Disorders of the TMJ. Oral and Maxillofacial Surgery Clinics North America. Philadelphia: Saunders; 1989.

TREATMENT

The treatment of TMJ osteoarthrosis and internal derangement can be divided into 3 broad categories: noninvasive, minimally invasive, and invasive management. The specific management plan can vary depending on the specific diagnosis and severity of TMJ disorder; however, the underlying principles of treatment apply universally.

1. Multidisciplinary approach involving multiple specialties, including general dentistry, oral medicine, orofacial pain, orthodontics, oral surgery, physical therapy, and psychiatry may be necessary to fully address the problem from all angles.
2. There is progression of treatment only after failure of more conservative modalities. The least invasive and most reversible treatments should be tried first. Only after a

failure to alter the disease process and clinical symptoms should more invasive and often nonreversible treatments be initiated.

Goals of treatment
1. Decreasing joint pain
2. Increasing joint function and opening
3. Preventing further joint damage
4. Improving overall quality of life and reducing disease-related morbidities

NONINVASIVE TREATMENT OPTIONS
Occlusal or Stabilization Splints

Physicians have used various types of splints since the eighteenth century for the treatment of TMJ disorders.[22] Today the use of splints has become one of the most common in office initial treatments for TMD-associated pain. Since their inception, splints are thought to work by unloading the condyle and in effect protecting the TMJ and articular disk from degeneration and excessive articular strain.[22] Although there are varying designs, they all function similarly to disengage the condylar head from the fossa and articular disk (see **Table 1**).

A recent meta-analysis of randomized controlled trials evaluating intraoral orthopedic appliances for TMD showed that hard stabilization appliances have good evidence of modest efficacy in the treatment of temporomandibular joint dysfunction (TMJD) pain compared with nonoccluding appliances and no treatment. Other types of appliances, including soft stabilization appliances, anterior positioning appliances, and anterior bite appliances, have some evidence of efficacy in reducing TMD pain.[23] However, a Cochrane Database review of stabilization splint therapy for TMJ pain revealed that there is insufficient evidence either for or against the use of stabilization splint therapy.[24] Clearly further randomized controlled studies with larger sample sizes and longer duration of follow-up are needed to study the effectiveness of splint therapy for TMD pain (**Table 2**).

Pharmacotherapy

Pharmacologic therapy in conjunction with other treatment modalities often plays an important role in the management of articular disk and TMJ disorders. The aim of pharmacotherapy can be divided into 2 main goals[25]:

1. Treatment of the underlying disease process
2. Alleviation of disease associated symptoms, such as pain and swelling

There are various classes of medications that function to target each of the 2 treatment goals (see **Box 1**). Oftentimes it is necessary to use a combination of medications to treat both the pain as well as the inflammatory disease process, depending

Table 2	
Major types of occlusal splints used in TMD therapy	
Splint Type	**Design**
Stabilization splint	Hard acrylic with full coverage of maxillary and mandibular dentition in centric occlusion
Repositioning splint	Hard acrylic with full coverage of maxillary or mandibular dentition with inclines to guide mandible to a more anterior position
Soft splint	Similar to hard stabilization splints but made from a more inexpensive pliable material

on the severity of disease. However, care must be taken to avoid the prolonged use of certain medications, in particular analgesics, to prevent drug tolerance and dependency. The health provider's ultimate goal should be symptomatic relief for a period of time in the hopes that this will break the disease cycle and lead to permanent improvement.

Despite the frequent use of pharmacologic agents, numerous review articles have shown insufficient evidence to support or not support the effectiveness of pharmacologic interventions for pain in patients with TMJ disorders.[26,27] There is an obvious need for further randomized controlled trials to study the effectiveness of pharmacologic interventions to treat pain associated with TMD (**Table 3**).

Physical Therapy

Physical therapy is commonly used in the outpatient setting to relieve musculoskeletal pain, reduce inflammation, and restore oral motor function. Physical therapy plays an adjunctive role in virtually all TMJ disorders treatment regimens. Various physical therapy modalities are available to the outpatient health provider (see **Table 2**). Although the evidence is weak, there are numerous systematic review articles that support the efficacy of exercise therapy, thermal therapy, and acupuncture to reduce symptoms, such as pain, swelling, and TMJ hypomobility (**Table 4**).[29-31]

MINIMALLY INVASIVE TREATMENT OPTIONS
Intra-articular Injections

Different therapeutic solutions can be injected directly into the TMJ space and allow for the targeted treatment of inflammation and joint degeneration (see **Table 3**). The TMJ has 2 unconnected cavities, superior and inferior, partitioned by the articular disk. The superior space injection is the commonly used technique. However, a recent review article showed that an inferior space injection, or simultaneous upper and lower spaces injections, seemed to be more effective with increasing mouth opening and decreasing TMJ-associated pain (**Table 5**).[35]

Table 3 Types of medication used in TMD treatment		
Class	**Examples**	**Function**
NSAIDs	Ibuprofen, naproxen, diclofenac, aspirin, etodolac	Reduce inflammation and pain
Opioids	Codeine, oxycodone, morphine, hydromorphone, meperidine	Reduce pain
Corticosteroids	Prednisone, dexamethasone, hydrocortisone	Reduce inflammation and pain
Muscle relaxants	Cyclobenzaprine, carisoprodol, baclofen	Reduce muscle spasm
Antidepressants	Amitriptyline, trazodone, fluoxetine, sertraline	Reduce muscle tension
Anxiolytics	Alprazolam, lorazepam, oxazepam, diazepam, buspirone	Reduce tension and muscle spasm

Abbreviation: NSAIDs, nonsteroidal antiinflammatory drugs.
Data from List T, Axelsson S, Leijon G. Pharmacologic interventions in the treatment of temporomandibular disorders, atypical facial pain, and burning mouth syndrome. A qualitative systematic review. J Orofac Pain 2003;17(4):301–10.

Table 4 Description of treatment modalities for articular disk and TMJ osteroarthrosis	
Modality	**Description**
Exercise therapy	Techniques include manual therapy, postural exercises, muscle stretching, and strengthening exercises.[28] Passive and active stretching of muscles or range-of-motion exercise are performed to increase oral opening and decrease pain.[28]
Thermal therapy	It involves the superficial application of a dry or moist heat/cold pad directly to the affected area typically in 20-min intervals. It is used in conjunction with exercise therapy in the treatment of inflammation and TMJ hypomobility.
Acupuncture	It is thought to stimulate the production of endorphins, serotonin, and acetylcholine within the central nervous system, or it may relieve pain by acting as a noxious stimulus. Treatments involve placement of needles in the face and hands and are typically given weekly for a total of 6 wk.[29]

Arthrocentesis/Arthroscopy

Arthrocentesis and arthroscopy are safe and quick minimally invasive procedures that are used in patients who are resistant to more conservative treatment modalities. Oftentimes they are combined with immediate postoperative intra-articular injections and the use of occlusal splints, pharmacotherapy, and physical therapy during the recovery period (**Tables 6** and **7**).[38]

INVASIVE TREATMENT OPTIONS
Arthroplasty

TMJ arthroplasty involves the reshaping of the articular surface to remove osteo-phytes, erosions, and irregularities found in osteoarthritis refractory to other treatment modalities.[34] These patients frequently also present with articular disk degeneration or displacement, which can be repositioned, repaired, or entirely removed. All such procedures should be performed by an experienced oral surgeon under general anesthesia, and this is done using an open surgical approach through a periauricular

Table 5 Types of intra-articular injections used in treatment of TMJ and articular disk disorders		
	Hyaluronic Acid	**Corticosteroids**
Benefits	A natural component of TMJ synovial fluid and lubricates and maintains the normal internal environment of the joints[32]	Reduction of inflammatory factors and reducing the activity of the immune system
Adverse effects	Mild pain and swelling at injection site, mostly transient[33]	Infection and destruction of articular cartilage; avoid long-term repeat injections[34]
Efficacy	Improved long-term clinical signs of TMD and overall improvement of symptoms in comparison with placebo; no difference in radiological progression of disease[32]	Same short-term and long-term improvements in symptoms, clinical signs, and overall condition compared with hyaluronic acid[32]

Table 6 Arthrocentesis for TMD treatment	Arthrocentesis
Description	Saline lavage of the superior joint space, hydraulic pressure and manipulation to release adhesions, and elimination of intra-articular inflammatory mediators (**Fig. 3**)[36,37]; less invasive than arthroscopy and can be done in outpatient setting with local anesthesia and intravenous sedation
Indication	• Limited opening with anteriorly displaced articular disk without reduction • Chronic pain with good range of movement and displaced articular disk with reduction • Degenerative osteoarthritis
Contraindications	• TMJ with bony or fibrous ankylosis • Extracapsular source of pain • Patients who have not undergone noninvasive treatment modalities
Efficacy	Recently reported 83.5% treatment success rate in patients with internal derangement and osteoarthritis (as defined as an improvement in maximum jaw opening and a reduction in pain level and mandibular dysfunction)[38]

Data from Fonseca RJ. Oral and maxillofacial surgery. Chicago: Saunders; 2000.

skin incision (**Fig. 5**). Complications are rare but can include wound infection, facial nerve injury, permanent occlusal changes, relapsing joint pain, and life-threatening vascular injuries.[42] As with all TMJ-related surgeries, early postoperative physical therapy and range-of-motion exercises are vital to achieving long-term functional improvements.

- Disk repositioning: Reposition the disk back to its normal anatomic position in patients with internal derangement. This procedure is most effective in disks that are normal appearing (white, firm, shiny) with minimal displacement.
- Disk repair: Small disk perforations can be repaired with a tension-free primary closure.
- Discectomy alone: Removal of the articular disk is indicated in patients with severe disk perforation, complete loss of disk elasticity, and who are persistently symptomatic even after disk repositioning.[43] Although studies have shown there

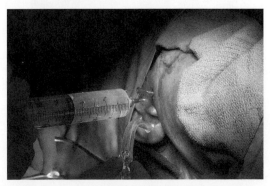

Fig. 3. Minimally invasive treatment of TMD: Arthrocentesis.

Table 7 Arthroscopy for TMD treatment	
	Arthroscopy
Description	Involves insertion of an arthroscope and inspection of the TMJ under fluid distention under general anesthesia; allows for irrigation of joint space, lysis of these adhesions, and mobilization of the joint under direct visualization[39] **(Fig. 4)**
Indication	• Limited opening and pain secondary to internal derangement • TMJ hypomobility secondary to fibrosis or adhesions • Degenerative osteoarthritis
Contraindications	• TMJ with severe bony or fibrous ankylosis • Extracapsular source of pain • Patients who have not undergone noninvasive treatment modalities • Practitioner with lack of open joint surgery experience
Efficacy	A large multicenter study reports more than 90% success rate as defined as improved mobility, pain, and function.[40] Arthroscopy led to greater improvement in opening after 12 mo than arthrocentesis; however, there was no difference in pain.[41]

Data from Fonseca RJ. Oral and Maxillofacial Surgery. Chicago: Saunders; 2000.

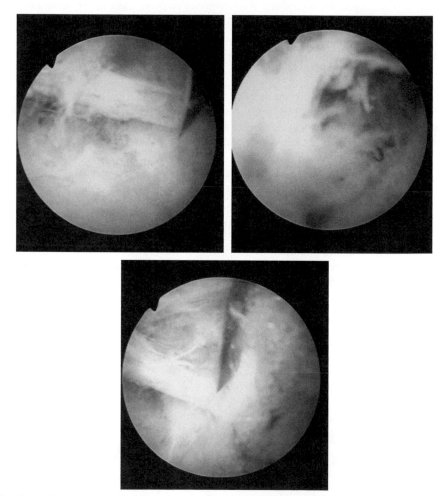

Fig. 4. Arthroscopic view of temporomandibular joint space showing evidence of multiple disk adhensions.

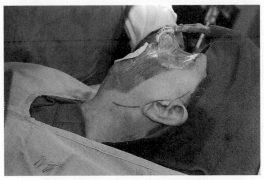

Fig. 5. Open surgical approach made through outlined periauricular and endural skin incision.

is generally an improvement in pain and maximal mouth opening following the surgical removal of the disk, patients also exhibited signs of fibrous adhesions, narrowing of joint space, and osteophyte formation on MRI.[44–46]

- Discectomy with graft replacement: The placement of a graft is thought to protect the joint from further degeneration and prevent the formation of fibrous adhesions. The use of autogenous sources, such as temporalis flaps, auricular cartilage, and dermal grafts, results in superior clinical outcomes compared with alloplastic grafts.[42] Studies have showed that autogenous grafts actually did not prevent remodeling of the joint but may help to reduce the onset of crepitus resulting from discectomy alone.[47,48] However, it was shown that discectomy with dermis graft replacement does result in a statistically significant improvement in pain, chewing, and general health (**Box 2**).

Total Joint Replacement

TMJ replacement is intended primarily at restoration of form and function, and any pain relief gained is only a secondary benefit.[47] The need for TMJ replacement typically indicates severely damaged joints with end-stage disease that has failed all other more conservative treatment modalities. Autogenous costochondral bone grafts have been frequently used in TMJ reconstruction in the past because of its gross anatomic similarity to the mandibular condyle, ease of adaptation to the recipient site, and its demonstrated growth potential in juveniles.[49] However, because of potential harvest-site morbidity and failure during the transplantation process or from functional

---

Box 2
Criteria for successful TMJ disk surgery

1. Mild, brief pain of no concern to patients

2. Vertical range of motion greater than 35 mm and lateral range of motion greater than 6 mm

3. Ability to tolerate a regular diet

4. Stabilization of any degenerative radiological changes

5. Absence of symptoms for at least 2 years

6. Absence of significant surgical complications

Data from Holmlund AB. Surgery for TMJ internal derangement. Evaluation of treatment and criteria for success. Int J Oral Maxillofac Surg 1993;22:75–7.

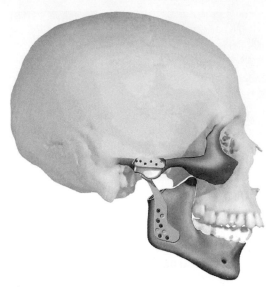

Fig. 6. Total joint replacement consisting of a fossa and condylar component held in place by screw fixation.

loading, the use of alloplastic materials has become increasingly more popular in the adult population.[42] Currently, various custom and stock titanium joint designs are available, which consist of both a fossa and a condylar component held in place by screw fixation (**Fig. 6**). Studies have shown that both custom and stock alloplastic

---

Box 3
Indications and relative contraindications for TMJ alloplastic replacement

Indications

1. Ankylosis or reankylosis with severe anatomic abnormalities

2. Failure of autogenous grafts in patients who underwent multiple operations

3. Destruction of autogenous graft tissue by pathosis

4. Severe inflammatory joint disease that results in anatomic mutilation of the total joint components and functional disability

5. Failure of Proplast-Teflon implant (Vitek Inc, Houston, Texas)

6. Failure of Vitek-Kent total or partial joints (Vitek, Inc, Houston, Texas)

Relative contraindications

1. Pediatric patients with immature facial skeleton

2. Patients with unrealistic expectations or lack of understanding of procedure

3. Uncontrolled systemic disease

4. Allergy to implant material

5. Active infection at implantation site

Data from Dimitroulis G. A critical review of interpositional grafts following temporomandibular joint discectomy with an overview of the dermis-fat graft. Int J Oral Maxillofac Surg 2011;40:561–8.

TMJ replacements resulted in statistically significant improvement in pain level, jaw function, and incisal opening (**Box 3**).[50,51]

REFERENCES

1. Wadhwa S, Kapila S. TMJ Disorders: future innovations in diagnostics and therapeutics. J Dent Educ 2008;72(8):930–47.
2. Ghali GE, Miloro M, Waite PD, et al, editors. Peterson's principles of oral and maxillofacial surgery. 3rd edition. Shelton (CT): Pmph USA; 2012.
3. Lipton JA, Ship JA, Larach-Robinson D. Estimated prevalence and distribution of reported orofacial pain in the United States. J Am Dent Assoc 1993;124: 115–21.
4. Manfredini D, Guarda-Nardini L, Winocur E, et al. Research diagnostic criteria for temporomandibular disorders: a systematic review of axis I epidemiologic findings. Oral Surg Oral Med Oral Pathol Oral Radiol Endod 2011;112: 453–62.
5. Abubaker AO, Raslan WF, Sotereanos GC. Estrogen and progesterone receptors in temporomandibular joint discs of symptomatic and asymptomatic persons: a preliminary study. J Oral Maxillofac Surg 1993;51:1096–100.
6. Milam SB, Aufdemorte TB, Sheridan PJ, et al. Sexual dimorphism in the distribution of estrogen receptors in the temporomandibular joint complex of the baboon. Oral Surg Oral Med Oral Pathol 1987;64:527–32.
7. Aufdemorte TB, Van Sickels JE, Dolwick MF, et al. Estrogen receptors in the temporomandibular joint of the baboon (Papio cynocephalus): an autoradiographic study. Oral Surg Oral Med Oral Pathol 1986;61:307–14.
8. Mohlin B, Kopp S. A clinical study on the relationship between malocclusion, occlusal interferences, and mandibular pain and dysfunction. Swed Dent J 1978;2:103.
9. Perry H. Relationship of the occlusion to temporomandibular joint dysfunction. A retrospective study. J Prosthet Dent 1977;39:420.
10. Upton L, Scott R, Haywood J. Major maxillomandibular malrelations and temporomandibular joint pain-dysfunction. J Prosthet Dent 1984;51:686.
11. Williamson E. Temporomandibular dysfunction in pretreatment adolescence patients. Am J Orthod 1977;72:429.
12. Riolo M, Brandt D, Tenhaue T. Association between occlusal characteristics and signs and symptoms of TMJ dysfunction in children and young adults. Am J Orthod Dentofacial Orthop 1987;92:467.
13. Rasmussen O. Description of population and progress of symptoms in a longitudinal study of temporomandibular joint arthropathy. Scand J Dent Res 1981; 89:196–203.
14. McNeill C. Temporomandibular disorders: guidelines for classification, assessment, and management. The American Academy of orofacial pain. Chicago: Quintessence; 1993.
15. Blankestijn J, Boering G. Posterior dislocation of the temporomandibular disc. Int J Oral Surg 1985;14:437–43.
16. Liedberg J, Westesson P, Kurita K. Side-ways and rotational displacement of the temporomandibular joint disk: diagnosis by arthrography and correlation to cryosectional morphology. Oral Surg Oral Med Oral Pathol 1990;69: 757–63.
17. Sanders B. Management of internal derangements of the temporomandibular joint. Semin Orthod 1995;4(1):244–57.

18. Tallents RH, Katzberg RW, Murphy W, et al. Magnetic resonance imaging findings in asymptomatic volunteers and symptomatic patients with temporomandibular disorders. J Prosthet Dent 1996;75:529.

19. Wilkes C. Internal derangement of the temporomandibular joint. In: Clark G, Sanders B, Bertolami C, editors. Advances in diagnostic and surgical arthroscopy of the temporomandibular joint. Philadelphia: Sanders; 1993.

20. Dworkin SF, Leresche L. Research diagnostic criteria for temporomandibular disorders: review, criteria, examinations and specifications, critique. J Craniomandib Disord 1992;6:301–55.

21. Shaefer J, Riley C, Caruso P, et al. Analysis of criteria for MRI diagnosis of TMJ disc displacement and arthralgia. Int J Dent 2012;2012:283163.

22. Klasser GD, Greene CS. Oral appliances in the management of temporomandibular disorders. Oral Surg Oral Med Oral Pathol Oral Radiol Endod 2009; 107(2):212–23.

23. Fricton J, Look JO, Wright E, et al. Systematic review and meta-analysis of randomized controlled trials evaluating intraoral orthopedic appliances for temporomandibular disorders. J Orofac Pain 2010;24(3):237–54.

24. Al-Ani MZ, Davies SJ, Gray RJ, et al. Stabilisation splint therapy for temporomandibular pain dysfunction syndrome. Cochrane Database Syst Rev 2004;(1):CD002778.

25. Dionne RA. Pharmacologic treatments for temporomandibular disorders. Oral Surg Oral Med Oral Pathol Oral Radiol Endod 1997;83(1):134 42.

26. Mujakperuo HR, Watson M, Morrison R, et al. Pharmacological interventions for pain in patients with temporomandibular disorders. Cochrane Database Syst Rev 2010;(10):CD004715.

27. List T, Axelsson S, Leijon G. Pharmacologic interventions in the treatment of temporomandibular disorders, atypical facial pain, and burning mouth syndrome. A qualitative systematic review. J Orofac Pain 2003;17(4):301–10.

28. Fricton JR. Management of masticatory myofascial pain. Semin Orthod 1995; 1(4):229–43.

29. Rosted P. Practical recommendations for the use of acupuncture in the treatment of temporomandibular disorders based on the outcome of published controlled studies. Oral Dis 2001;7(2):109–15.

30. McNeely ML, Armijo Olivo S, Magee DJ. A systematic review of the effectiveness of physical therapy interventions for temporomandibular disorders. Phys Ther 2006;86(5):710–25.

31. Cho SH, Whang WW. Acupuncture for temporomandibular disorders: a systematic review. J Orofac Pain 2010;24(2):152–62.

32. Shi Z, Guo C, Awad M. Hyaluronate for temporomandibular joint disorders [review]. Cochrane Database Syst Rev 2003;(1):CD002970.

33. Bertolami CN, Gay T, Clark GT, et al. Use of sodium hyaluronate in treating temporomandibular joint disorders: a randomized, double blind, placebo controlled clinical trial. J Oral Maxillofac Surg 1993;51:232–42.

34. Tanaka E, Detamore MS, Mercuri LG. Degenerative disorders of the temporomandibular joint: etiology, diagnosis, and treatment. J Dent Res 2008;87: 296.

35. Li C, Zhang Y, Lv J, et al. Inferior or double joint spaces injection versus superior joint space injection for temporomandibular disorders: a systematic review and meta-analysis. J Oral Maxillofac Surg 2012;70(1):37–44.

36. Guo C, Shi Z, Revington P. Arthrocentesis and lavage for treating temporomandibular joint disorders. Cochrane Database Syst Rev 2009;(4):CD004973.

37. Nitzan DW. Arthrocentesis for management of severe closed lock of the tempo-romandibular joint. Oral Maxillofac Surg Clin North Am 1994;6:245–57.
38. Monje-Gil F, Nitzan D, González-Garcia R. Temporomandibular joint arthrocent-esis. Review of the literature. Med Oral Patol Oral Cir Bucal 2012;17(4):e575–81.
39. Indresano AT. Surgical arthroscopy as the preferred treatment for internal derangements of the temporomandibular joint. J Oral Maxillofac Surg 2001; 59(3):308–12.
40. McCain JP, Sanders B, Koslin MG, et al. Temporomandibular joint arthroscopy: a 6-year multicenter retrospective study of 4,831 joints. J Oral Maxillofac Surg 1992;50(9):926–30.
41. Rigon M, Pereira LM, Bortoluzzi MC, et al. Arthroscopy for temporomandibular disorders. Cochrane Database Syst Rev 2011;(5):CD006385.
42. Fonseca RJ. Oral and maxillofacial surgery. Chicago: Saunders; 2000. Print.
43. Lanz AB. Discitis mandibularis. Zentralbl Chir 1909;36:289–91.
44. Westesson PL, Cohen JM, Tallents RH. Magnetic-resonance-imaging of temporomandibular-joint after surgical-treatment of internal derangement. Oral Surg Oral Med Oral Pathol 1991;71:407–11.
45. Hansson LG, Eriksson L, Westesson PL. Magnetic-resonance evaluation after temporomandibular-joint discectomy. Oral Surg Oral Med Oral Pathol 1992;74: 801–10.
46. Miloro M, Henriksen B. Discectomy as the primary surgical option for internal derangement of the temporomandibular joint. J Oral Maxillofac Surg 2010;68: 782–9.
47. Dimitroulis G. A critical review of interpositional grafts following temporomandib-ular joint discectomy with an overview of the dermis-fat graft. Int J Oral Maxillo-fac Surg 2011;40:561–8.
48. Mercuri LG. Alloplastic temporomandibular joint reconstruction. Oral Surg Oral Med Oral Pathol Oral Radiol Endod 1998;85:631–7.
49. MacIntosh RB. The use of autogenous tissue in temporomandibular joint recon-struction. J Oral Maxillofac Surg 2000;58:63–9.
50. Wolford LM, Pitta MC, Reiche-Fischel O, et al. TMJ Concepts/Techmedica custom-made TMJ total joint prosthesis: 5-year follow-up study. Int J Oral Max-illofac Surg 2003;32(3):268–74.
51. Giannakopoulos HE, Sinn DP, Quinn PD. Biomet Microfixation Temporomandib-ular Joint Replacement System: a 3-year follow-up study of patients treated during 1995 to 2005. J Oral Maxillofac Surg 2012;70(4):787–94.

Cranial Neuralgias

Wendy S. Hupp, DMD*, F. John Firriolo, DDS, PhD

KEYWORDS

- Trigeminal neuralgia • Glossopharyngeal neuralgia • Nervus intermedius neuralgia
- Postherpetic neuralgia • Clinical findings

KEY POINTS

- Cranial neuralgias are uncommon, localized, excruciating pains in the orofacial region.
- History is the most important information to diagnose these disorders.
- Anticonvulsant medications are the first line of therapy; surgical treatment can also be successful.
- Postherpetic neuralgia occurs secondary to recurrent herpes zoster and may persist for months to years.
- Prevention is the best way to avoid postherpetic neuralgia.

The cranial neuralgias that will be discussed here include several types of conditions that are related by the location of the pain in the face and head and that the cause of the pain is from the sensory nerve tissue within that area. Also known as neuropathic or neurogenic, these conditions include structural and/or functional abnormalities in the peripheral or central nervous system (CNS).[1] The nerve abnormality may be caused by infection, trauma, metabolic abnormalities, chemotherapy, surgery, radiation, neurotoxins, compression, inflammation, or tumor infiltration. Dentists may be asked to help determine if there is an odontogenic cause to the pain and also may be called on to refer patients to the appropriate specialist for further testing.

Typical characteristics of cranial neuralgia pain are described as electric shocklike or lancinating. It is almost always unilateral, although approximately 3% to 5% of cases occur bilaterally. Patients have a period without pain or even slight paresthesia after the attack.[2]

There are 2 broad categories of cranial neuralgias: those that have episodic symptoms and those that produce continuous symptoms. The episodic or paroxysmal attacks last seconds to minutes, and may be frequent or separated by long periods

Disclosures: None.
Conflict of Interest: None.
Department of General Dentistry and Oral Medicine, School of Dentistry, University of Louisville, 501 South Preston Street, Louisville, KY 40292, USA
* Corresponding author.
E-mail address: wendy.hupp@louisville.edu

Dent Clin N Am 57 (2013) 481–495
http://dx.doi.org/10.1016/j.cden.2013.04.009
0011-8532/13/$ – see front matter © 2013 Elsevier Inc. All rights reserved.

dental.theclinics.com

Definitions related to neuralgias

Allodynia is pain resulting from a non-noxious stimulus (ie, a stimulus that normally does not cause pain).

Dysesthesia is an abnormal or unpleasant sensation (eg, burning, stinging, or stabbing).

Hyperalgesia is an exaggerated or increased response to painful stimuli.

Hyperpathia is an exaggerated pain response whereby slightly painful stimulus is perceived as painful.

Paresthesia is an abnormal but not always unpleasant sensation (eg, heaviness, tingling, or numbness).

Refractory period is when the nerve tissue is unable to propagate an impulse, no sensation is noted, and there are pain-free intervals of varying duration.

---

of time of remission. Often there is a triggering event, such as a superficial, delicate touch to the face or mouth. The area of pain precisely follows the area enervated by a specific nerve. For some patients, the pain is excruciating and incapacitating, and they suffer other comorbid problems, such as anxiety and depression. Expeditious treatment is important to improve patients' quality of life; the sooner these neuralgias are treated, the better the prognosis. There is also a correlation with underlying compressive or inflammatory disease that must be examined.[3,4]

Some patients with continuous pain report a varying intensity of dull aching, burning, or throbbing that is punctuated by sharp pains. These patients do not have periods of total remission.[1] For many patients, the continuous pain is often misdiagnosed as a toothache or headache.

Cranial neuralgias that are characterized by both episodic and continuous pain in the orofacial region are described in this article. The International Headache Society (IHS)[5] has classified these cranial neuralgias as shown in **Box 1**. Postherpetic neuralgia is also discussed.

CLINICAL FINDINGS OF CRANIAL NEURALGIAS
Trigeminal Neuralgia

Trigeminal neuralgia (TN) is the most common of the cranial nerve neuralgias. There are estimates of 5 to 12 cases per 100,000 people in the United States, with a slight female predilection. TN can occur at any age, with 90% of patients aged more than 40 years; the peak patient age is 50 to 60 years. The right side is more commonly affected than the left.[6] It is not likely to have a familial pattern.[2,6] TN is also called *tic douloureux,* which is French for painful spasm. It has been known for hundreds of years as one of the most painful conditions experienced by man. The neuralgia affects the somatic sensory branches of the trigeminal nerve, but patients may have muscle contractions of the face in response to the paroxysms of pain.[1]

Classic TN (also called idiopathic or primary TN)[7] usually affects the second or third division of the trigeminal nerve, affecting the cheek or chin on one side. There is a sharp, stabbing pain with a sudden onset that can last less than a second to a few seconds, sometimes in a cluster of variable intensity up to 2 minutes.[6] It may be followed by a brief refractory period. The trigger may be a light touch on the skin, eating, shaving, washing, applying makeup, brushing of teeth, movement of the jaw or tongue, or a thermal stimulus.

Some patients with classic TN may have a progression to 2 or all 3 divisions of the trigeminal nerve over time, but the first (ophthalmic) division is involved alone in only

---

Box 1
IHS classification of cranial neuralgias and central causes of facial pain

13.1 Trigeminal neuralgia

    13.1.1 Classic trigeminal neuralgia

    13.1.2 Symptomatic trigeminal neuralgia

13.2 Glossopharyngeal neuralgia

    13.2.1 Classic glossopharyngeal neuralgia

    13.2.2 Symptomatic glossopharyngeal neuralgia

13.3 Nervus intermedius neuralgia

13.4 Superior laryngeal neuralgia

13.5 Nasociliary neuralgia

13.6 Supraorbital neuralgia

13.7 Other terminal branch neuralgias

13.8 Occipital neuralgia

Data from Headache Classifications Subcommittee of the International Headache Society. The international classification of headache disorders, 2nd edition. Cephalalgia 2004;24(Suppl 1): 9–160.

5% of reported cases.[6] About 35% have division II and division III involvement simultaneously.[8] About 85% of patients with TN have classic TN.[7,8]

Symptomatic TN is similar in clinical findings to classical TN; however, patients have a clearly defined specific cause, such as a central nervous system tumor, trauma, or systemic disease[7] other than a nerve-vessel conflict leading to compression of the nerve.[6,9]

Some investigators describe atypical TN as a separate diagnosis in perhaps as many as 30% of cases.[7,8,10] These patients suffer the classic severe electric-shock pain that is short lasting; however, there is a background burning that continues in between the attacks. This dull pain is exceptionally resistant to medical treatment and has been theorized to be a worsening of classic TN, although the age of patients who have been diagnosed with atypical TN does not seem to be older than those with classic TN.[10]

Patients with multiple sclerosis (MS) are also susceptible to TN and may make up about 3% of the overall number of cases.[1,6,8,9] TN occurs in 1% to 5% of patients with MS, and they have approximately 20 times the prevalence of TN as compared with the general populace. Most patients with bilateral TN have MS.[1]

Glossopharyngeal Neuralgia

The glossopharyngeal nerve enervates the oropharynx, throat, base of the tongue, tonsillar fossa, and tympanic plexus. Glossopharyngeal neuralgia (GN) is "milder disease than trigeminal neuralgia"[2,4] with an incidence of 0.7 cases per 100,000 and an equal distribution between men and women. The pain is often described as a deep stabbing pain on one side of the throat that is sudden in onset. The pain may radiate to the tongue or tonsil area or to the ear. The attacks tend to last 8 to 50 seconds but may be longer[2] and may occur in clusters from weeks to months. A refractory period is common.

GN may be triggered by swallowing, chewing, talking, coughing, yawning, or turning the head; some patients will stop eating or drinking to avoid an attack.[1,2] It is occasionally accompanied by cardiovascular symptoms caused by crossover with the vagus nerve, such as bradycardia, asystole, hypotension, or syncope.[1,2,8] This condition is called vagoglossopharyngeal neuralgia.[11]

Patients with GN may be misdiagnosed with temporomandibular joint disorders, ear or sinus infections, or dental pain. Occasionally, patients may have GN and TN at the same time, which should lead to an examination for a CNS lesion.[1] A case report was published that described bilateral Eagle syndrome (the elongation of the styloid processes) as the cause of bilateral GN.[12]

Nervus Intermedius Neuralgia

The nervus intermedius is the sensory branch of the facial nerve that enervates the external auditory meatus, pinna of the ear, and some of the skin below the ear lobe. Nervus intermedius neuralgia (NIN) is also know as geniculate neuralgia; the pain is typically centered directly deep in the auditory canal of the ear, the external structures of the ear, the palate, tongue, or deeply in the facial musculature.[1,2] Rarely, the anterior two-thirds of the tongue and soft palate are also involved as triggers and/or sites of pain because of the afferent fibers of the facial nerve to these areas.[1]

NIN is rare and always unilateral.[2] The trigger may be swallowing, talking, or stimulation of the ear canal. Pain is sometimes misdiagnosed as headache, such as migraine, but NIN can be associated with tearing, salivation, bitter taste, tinnitus, or vertigo on the unilateral side.[2] Association with herpes zoster and NIN is not uncommon.[1,2]

Superior Laryngeal Neuralgia

The superior laryngeal nerve is a sensory branch of the vagus nerve that innervates the cricothyroid muscles and the vocal cords. In this neuralgia, the pain is paroxysmal and shocklike as in TN but may vary in intensity over seconds to minutes in the side of the thyroid cartilage, pyriform sinus, or angle of the jaw. If the auricular branch is also involved, the pain may extend to the posterior auricular region, shoulder, upper thorax, or palate.[1,2]

The triggers include talking, swallowing, yawning, coughing, turning the head, or straining the voice. Sometimes patients may report an urge to swallow.[1]

Occipital and Other Branch Neuralgias

The somatic sensory branches of the cervical spinal nerves may have similar neuralgias as the cranial nerves to the areas that they enervate. Patients with sudden, unilateral pains in the back of the head or neck should be evaluated for these problems that may confuse the clinician who is attempting to diagnose cervical or temporomandibular pain. Trigger points may include innocuous stimuli to the occipital region of the back of the head, neck, and shoulder muscles.

PATHOPHYSIOLOGY OF CRANIAL NEURALGIAS

There are several theories for the cause of cranial neuralgias. Many investigators report that the nerve or ganglion of a cranial nerve can be compressed by a blood vessel in close proximity to the nerve. This condition is also called a nerve-vessel conflict or neurovascular conflict. The pressure on the nerve may lead to a visible groove,[7] possibly leading to a loss of myelination. Because some axons are stimulated by innocuous stimuli, the electrical impulses can jump to adjacent, faster fibers that send the electrical shocklike message to the brain.

Another theory suggests that there is peripheral damage that leads to a paroxysmal discharge of the nerve that could lead to a reverberation of pain impulses along the track of the nerve.[2,9] These injured neurons may actually show ectopic discharges[7] and lead to changes in the CNS and inhibitory controls.[3,7]

Furthermore, it is postulated that damaged neurons may heal with alterations to the myelin that lead to extra sodium channels in the axonal cell membranes, which may help explain the efficacy of antiepileptic drugs that stabilize cell membranes.[9]

In TN, the Gasserian ganglion and the nerve roots of the trigeminal nerve may be affected by vessel pressure, usually the superior cerebellar artery[6] in the posterior cranial fossa. For GN, the compression may occur by the posterior inferior cerebellar artery as the glossopharyngeal nerve exits from the medulla before the jugular foramen and close to the vagus nerve. In NIN, the geniculate ganglion is sometimes the site of the compression, but the sensory branch of the facial nerve is close to the lateral edge of the pons[2] and may be compressed by the anterior inferior cerebellar artery.

Superior laryngeal neuralgia seems to occur when the internal branch of the superior laryngeal nerve is compressed by the thyrohyoid cartilage and/or the artery and vein that accompany the nerve through the foramen in the cartilage.[13] Occipital neuralgia and other cervical spinal neuralgias can be traced to the pressure on the nerve from muscle spasm, such as from the trapezius[14] or other muscles of the posterior neck. Whiplash injury and arthritic changes at the atlantoaxial joint are also implicated in causing the neuralgia.[15]

DIAGNOSIS OF CRANIAL NEURALGIAS

The diagnosis is largely based on patients' history (**Table 1**). It is important to differentiate odontogenic pain so that teeth are not removed or endodontically treated in error.[1] Eliciting and/or anesthetizing the trigger are helpful in the diagnostic process. Unfortunately, many patients are misdiagnosed as having a headache or temporomandibular pain. Most (90%) patients suffer for more than 1 year before the proper diagnosis is made[16] because there is no specific diagnostic test to confirm cranial neuralgias. For most patients with cranial neuralgias, there is no clinically evident neurologic deficit, although a refractory period following the paroxysmal pain may be experienced.

Magnetic resonance imaging and special radiographic studies may be helpful for finding space-occupying lesions of the CNS. However, neurologic mapping may appear normal, without anatomic abnormalities; but once the surgeon explores the area, a tortuous vessel may be discovered compressing the nerve.[7,11] In TN studies, some patients have no vascular contact to the trigeminal nerve when surgically exposed; in about 14% of cadavers, there was a compression noted, but there was no diagnosis of TN.[7]

TREATMENT MODALITIES

Pharmacotherapy is the first line of treatment of cranial neuralgias. The most successful medications are anticonvulsants, such as carbamazepine, oxcarbazepine, lamotrigine, pregabalin, gabapentin, and baclofen. These agents may be prescribed alone or in combination. There are significant side effects that may be limiting, such as sedation, dizziness, muscle weakness, cognitive impairment, dermatologic reactions, and bone marrow suppression.[17]

Table 1
Summary of important cranial neuralgias causing facial and/or head pain

	Clinical Presentation	ICHD-II Diagnostic Criteria[a]

Classic TN	It is characterized by paroxysmal, severe, intense pain that is almost always (95%–97%) unilateral and with a regional distribution limited to one or more divisions of the trigeminal nerve. It most commonly involves the second (maxillary) and third (mandibular) divisions, with the first (ophthalmic) division involved less than 5% of the time. The pain is frequently described as electric shocklike, lancinating, or shooting, with an abrupt onset and termination. Pain is commonly triggered by minimal stimuli (including washing, shaving, chewing, talking, brushing the teeth, and even cold wind/drafts) within the affected area. The duration of an attack usually ranges from a few seconds to 2 min and may be either isolated or repetitive at short intervals so that the individual attacks blend into one another. Between attacks, patients are usually asymptomatic; however, some patients report a burning or dull sensation, which tends to subside in time. Periods of remission from attacks, ranging from several months to years, occur in about 50% of patients.	A. There are paroxysmal attacks of pain lasting from a fraction of a second to 2 min, affecting one or more divisions of the trigeminal nerve.
		B. Pain has at least one of the following characteristics:
		  1. Intense, sharp, superficial, or stabbing
		  2. Precipitated from trigger areas or by trigger factors
		C. Attacks are stereotyped in individual patients.
		D. There is no clinically evident neurologic deficit.
		E. It is not attributed to another disorder.

Symptomatic TN	It is identical to classic TN except caused by a demonstrable structural lesion other than vascular compression.	*Criteria A, B, and C same as above* D. A causative lesion, other than vascular compression, has been demonstrated by special investigations and/or posterior fossa exploration.

Classic GN	It is characterized by paroxysmal, severe, lancinating, or electric shocklike pain that is almost always unilateral and with a regional distribution affecting the tonsillar fossa, posterior oropharynx, posterior region (base) of the tongue, auditory canal, or angle of the mandible. The painful attacks can be triggered by ordinary activity, including swallowing, speaking, laughing, coughing, sneezing, throat clearing, or rotation of the head. Occasionally a trigger zone is identified within the preauricular or postauricular area, the neck, or the external auditory canal. The duration of an attack usually ranges from less than 1 s up to 2 min but can sometimes occur in rapid and continuous succession. Bradycardia and syncope associated with an attack have been reported to occur in about 2% of patients.	A. There are paroxysmal attacks of facial pain lasting from a fraction of a second to 2 min and fulfilling criteria B and C.
		B. Pain has all of the following characteristics:
		  1. Unilateral location
		  2. Distribution within the posterior part of the tongue, tonsillar fossa, pharynx, or beneath the angle of the lower jaw and/or in the ear
		  3. Sharp, stabbing, and severe
		  4. Precipitated by swallowing, chewing, talking, coughing, and/or yawning
		C. Attacks are stereotyped in individual patients.
		D. There is no clinically evident neurologic deficit.
		E. It is not attributed to another disorder.

Symptomatic GN	It is identical to classic GN except an aching pain may persist between paroxysms, and sensory impairment may be found in the distribution of the glossopharyngeal nerve.	*Criteria A, B, and C same as above* D. A causative lesion has been demonstrated by special investigations and/or surgery.
Superior laryngeal neuralgia	It is characterized by severe, brief, paroxysmal pain radiating from the region of the hyoid bone to the lateral aspect of the throat, submandibular region (eg, horizontal ramus or angle of the mandible), and/or area under the earlobe. Pain is usually unilateral and is typically precipitated by swallowing or less frequently by straining the voice (eg, shouting) or turning the head. Pain may sometimes radiate to the posterior auricular region, shoulder, or palate. Pain usually can be triggered by pressure to the skin above and lateral to the thyroid cartilage where the internal branch of the superior laryngeal nerve pierces the thyrohyoid membrane.	A. There are pain paroxysms lasting for seconds or minutes in the throat, submandibular region, and/or under the ear and fulfilling criteria B–D. B. Paroxysms are triggered by swallowing, straining the voice, or head turning. C. A trigger point is present on the lateral aspect of the throat overlying the hypothyroid membrane. D. The condition is relieved by local anesthetic block and cured by section of the superior laryngeal nerve. E. It is not attributed to another disorder.

(continued on next page)

Table 1
(continued)

	Clinical Presentation	ICHD-II Diagnostic Criteria[a]
NIN (geniculate neuralgia, Hunt neuralgia)	It is typically characterized by brief paroxysms of severe, usually sharp or burning pain that is localized deeply in the auditory canal and radiates to the external auditory meatus. Additional symptoms, such as abnormal tearing and salivation, and taste disturbances (most frequently loss of taste), have sometimes been reported during occurrences. Symptoms are associated with a trigger zone in the posterior wall of the auditory canal.	A. There are pain paroxysms of intermittent occurrence, lasting for seconds or minutes, in the depth of the ear. B. There is presence of a trigger area in the posterior wall of the auditory canal. C. It is not attributed to another disorder.
Supraorbital neuralgia	It is most frequently characterized by episodic, often unilateral, long-lasting attacks of moderate to severe frontal pain in the region of the supraorbital notch and medial aspect of the forehead in the area supplied by the supraorbital nerve.	A. There is paroxysmal or constant pain in the region of the supraorbital notch and medial aspect of the forehead in the area supplied by the supraorbital nerve. B. There is tenderness over the nerve in the supraorbital notch. C. Pain is abolished by local anesthetic blockade or ablation of the supraorbital nerve.
Occipital neuralgia	It is characterized by paroxysmal shooting, stabbing, or jabbing pain at the base of the skull or neck that may radiate over the cranium and that follows the distribution of the greater, lesser, and/or third occipital nerve. Paroxysms can start spontaneously or may be provoked by specific actions, such as brushing the hair or moving the neck and rotation or lateral bending of the cervical spine. It is commonly associated with tenderness over the involved nerve and is sometimes accompanied by diminished sensation or dysesthesia in the affected area.	A. Paroxysmal stabbing pain, with or without persistent aching between paroxysms, in the distributions of the greater, lesser, and/or third occipital nerves. B. There is tenderness over the affected nerve. C. Pain is temporarily eased by local anesthetic block of the nerve.

| PHN | It is characterized by chronic pain persisting or recurring for 3 mo or more in the area affected by acute herpes zoster (ie, reactivation of varicella zoster virus infection). Herpes zoster affects the trigeminal ganglion in 8%–28% of patients, with isolated involvement of the ophthalmic division in about 80% of those patients. Approximately 10% of patients who have experienced herpes zoster involvement of the trigeminal nerve subsequently develop PHN. Spontaneous, constant, or intermittent pain may occur within the area of impaired or lost sensation and is frequently described as burning, throbbing, stabbing, shooting, or lancinating. Allodynia is reported in >70% of patients and most frequently occurs in areas with preserved sensation. The geniculate ganglion is rarely involved in PHN and may result in facial palsy, paralysis, and/or symptoms involving the auditory meatus. | A. There is head or facial pain in the distribution of a nerve or nerve division and fulfilling criteria C and D.
B. There is herpetic eruption in the territory of the same nerve.
C. The pain preceded herpetic eruption by <7 d.
D. Pain persists after 3 mo. |

Abbreviations: ICHD-II, International Classification of Headache Disorders, second edition; PHN, postherpetic neuralgia.

^a Headache Classification Subcommittee of the International Headache Society. The international classification of headache disorders, 2nd edition. Cephalalgia 2004;24(Suppl 1):9–160.

Further information concerning pharmacotherapy for cranial neuralgias is beyond the scope of this article, and the reader may wish to consult the cited references.[6,10,17,18]

Surgical treatment may be necessary for patients for whom the pharmacotherapy is unsuccessful and for patients who have nerve-vessel conflicts or other tumors. Microvascular decompression involves an open surgical approach through the cranium to expose the area of the vessel compression of the nerve. A barrier, such as Teflon (DuPont, Wilmington, DE, USA),[17] is placed between the nerve and blood vessel. Successful pain relief is found in up to 90% of patients initially, with 73% of patients pain free at 5 years.[6]

Other surgical techniques are considered destructive,[6,9] including rhizolysis using glycerol or alcohol, radiofrequency thermocoagulation, balloon decompression, and gamma knife procedures. Many of these patients will also show about 90% initial success; but at 5 years, pain returns in approximately 50%.[6] Gamma knife surgery is expensive, and initial pain relief may take up to 6 to 8 weeks.[19] The best results are when special neural imaging is used.[16]

Risks related to surgery include anesthesia, paresthesia, hemorrhage, aseptic meningitis, infection, cerebrospinal fluid leaks, and morbidity.[9,17] Risk of relapse increases with the severity of preoperative pain,[9] increased age, and prior surgery.[19]

CLINICAL FINDINGS OF POSTHERPETIC NEURALGIA

Following an initial (primary) varicella zoster virus (VZV) infection (chickenpox), the virus persists in a dormant (latent) state in the ganglia of sensory cranial nerves and spinal dorsal root ganglia and usually does not produce further symptoms for several decades. Reactivation of the dormant VZV virus is predominantly associated with an age-related decline in cell-mediated immunity and results in acute herpes zoster (HZ) (commonly known as shingles). HZ manifests as an acutely painful, red, maculopapular skin rash that evolves into vesicles, pustules, and crusts.[20,21] The skin rash of HZ follows a dermatomal distribution that generally corresponds to the area of skin innervated by a single spinal or cranial sensory ganglion; however, multiple (usually adjacent) dermatomes may be involved in approximately 20% of cases, especially in immunocompromised patients.[22] HZ has the highest incidence of all neurologic diseases, occurring annually in approximately 1 million people in the United States, with an incidence of 11.12 cases per 1000 patient-years in a sample of individuals aged 60 years or older.[23,24] In patients who are seropositive for antibodies to VZV, the overall lifetime risk of HZ is 10% to 20%, with approximately 50% of all cases of HZ occurring in patients older than 60 years, and the greatest incidence (30%) occurring in patients older than 80 years.[25,26] Symptoms of acute HZ typically resolve in about 2 to 4 weeks.

Postherpetic neuralgia (PHN) is the most common complication following an episode of acute HZ. Although there is no universally accepted definition of PHN, it is frequently defined as pain persisting or recurring in the area affected by HZ for 3 months or longer after the rash has healed.[22,27] PHN develops on average in 9% to 34% of persons with HZ depending on the definition of PHN used and the population studied. Because both the frequency and duration of PHN increase with age, the highest incidence of PHN (73%) has been reported to develop in adults with HZ who are 70 years of age or older.[20,24,27] The duration of symptomatic PHN is indefinite, and PHN has been reported to last more than 1 year in 20% of patients who are 60 years of age or older.[22,28]

The nerves most frequently affected by PHN seem to be the same as those that are most frequently affected by HZ. The thoracic dermatomes (especially T4–T6) are affected most frequently and are involved in up to 50% of patients with HZ.[29] These nerves are followed in frequency by the trigeminal nerve, which is affected in 8% to 28% of patients with HZ.[7] The cervical or lumbar dermatomes are involved in HZ in 10% to 20% of patients, and sacral dermatomes are affected in only 2% to 8% of persons.[29] The ophthalmic division of the trigeminal nerve is affected in more than 80% of those with trigeminal nerve HZ involvement; when this occurs, it is known as herpes zoster ophthalmicus (HZO).[20] HZO occurs in approximately 10% to 20% of patients with HZ and can involve the entire eye causing uveitis, scleritis, keratoconjunctivitis, optic neuritis; it may be complicated by secondary bacterial infection. HZO is usually painful; in some patients, it can result in permanent vision loss.[30,31] PHN occurs in about 10% of patients with HZO.[32,33]

Geniculate HZ (or Ramsay Hunt syndrome) is a localized HZ infection that affects the geniculate ganglion, vestibulocochlear nerve ganglion, and facial nerve. It is typically characterized by vesicles occurring on the pinna and in the external auditory canal along the distribution of the sensory branch of the facial nerve (HZ oticus), with transient or permanent vestibulocochlear dysfunction (ie, hearing loss, vertigo) and facial nerve palsy or paralysis. Less often, vesicular lesions also occur on the anterior pillar of the tonsillar fauces. The chorda tympani may also be affected, leading to loss of taste on the anterior two-thirds of the tongue.[32] Ramsay Hunt syndrome is a relatively rare disease affecting approximately 1 in 20,000 people.[34]

The risk of PHN seems to increase with age. A large population-based study by Yawn and colleagues[35] of 1669 adult patients with a confirmed diagnosis of HZ from 1996 through 2001 reported the rate of PHN (defined in this study as at least 90 days of documented pain) increased from 5% in those younger than 60 years to 10% in those aged 60 to 69 years and to 20% in those aged 80 years or older. Other factors that have been identified to significantly increase the risk for PHN are female sex, the presence of a prodrome (ie, pain and/or abnormal sensations before HZ rash onset), greater severity of the preceding HZ rash (ie, the number of papules, vesicles, or crusted vesicles), and greater acute pain severity of the preceding HZ rash.[25,36–39]

The pain experienced by patients with PHN may manifest in several different forms including allodynia (ordinary nonpainful stimulus that is perceived as painful), hyperpathia (an exaggerated pain response where slightly painful stimulus is perceived as painful), and dysesthesia (abnormal sensations are experienced in the absence of stimulation).[21,40] According to Johnson and colleagues,[22] patients with PHN describe characteristic patterns of pain, with the majority experiencing at least 2 of the following 3 patterns:

- Spontaneous, constant, deep burning, throbbing and aching pain
- Intermittent sharp, stabbing, shooting, lancinating pain, which may also be spontaneous
- Allodynia that usually lasts well beyond the duration of the stimulus

At least 70% to more than 90% of patients with PHN experience allodynia that tends to occur in areas where sensation is relatively preserved.[41] In contrast, patients with PHN tend to experience spontaneous pain in areas where sensation is lost or impaired.[42] Allodynia is frequently described as the most distressing and debilitating component of PHN and can sometimes be associated with clinical depression. Patients with mechanical allodynia experience severe pain after light, normally innocuous, mechanical stimulation of the affected area by things as minor as light touch of the skin by a brush or a piece of clothing as well as cold allodynia (eg, pain triggered by a cool breeze).[22] Additionally, thermal hyperalgesia (pain of exaggerated severity in response to normally painful thermal stimulation) has been reported in approximately one-third of patients experiencing PHN.[27] It is not uncommon for the pain of PHN to significantly interfere with routine daily activities and sleep, even with appropriate treatment.[20,22]

PATHOPHYSIOLOGY OF POSTHERPETIC NEURALGIA

The pathophysiology of PHN is complex and involves multiple, distinct processes within the peripheral nervous system and the CNS leading to neuropathic pain as a result of specific nerve fiber injury caused by the host immune response and inflammation that is triggered by the reactivation of VZV in HZ.[22,43]

For example, in PHN involving the trigeminal nerve, inflammatory changes and related nerve injury and/or dysfunction have been found throughout the peripheral and central trigeminal pathways and even as far caudal as the lower portion of the descending trigeminal tract in the cervical spinal cord.[32] A study by Truini and colleagues[44] of patients with trigeminal PHN provided evidence that the function of both nociceptive and well as non-nociceptive trigeminal never fibers were impaired. Specifically, it is thought that the constant pain seen in trigeminal PHN is caused by a marked loss of nociceptive afferent unmyelinated C nerve fibers, whereas paroxysmal pain is related to Aβ nerve fiber demyelination.

DIAGNOSIS OF POSTHERPETIC NEURALGIA

The diagnosis of PHN is usually made from patient history and distinctive clinical findings. A history of persistent ($\geq$3 months), unilateral, itching, burning, sharp, stabbing, or throbbing pain that is sufficiently intense to interfere with sleep and other normal daily activities and that is located in the dermatomes or adjoining area associated with a previous resolved HZ rash strongly supports the diagnosis of PHN. Additionally, areas affected by previous acute HZ may show evidence of cutaneous scarring.[29] However, PHN may occur months or even years after the resolution of HZ and patients may not remember the rash or associate the current pain with the prior episode of HZ.[45] Also, HZ is rarely known to occur as nerve pain in the absence of any skin rash or eruption (a condition known as zoster sine herpete) and may, therefore, confound or obscure the diagnosis of PHN.[46] In the event of a remote and/or subclinical episode of HZ, the presence of serum antibodies to HZ may help support a diagnosis of pain caused by PHN, especially if it occurs secondary to a case of zoster sine herpete.[27]

MANAGEMENT OF POSTHERPETIC NEURALGIA

Arguably, the most effective strategy for the management of PHN is its prevention. The HZ vaccine (zoster vaccine live [Zostavax], Merck, Whitehouse Station, NJ, USA) was initially approved for use by the US Food and Drug Administration (FDA) in May 2006 for people 60 years of age and older. In March 2011, the FDA expanded approval of the use of this vaccine in people aged 50 to 59 years. In the Shingles Prevention Study, the Zostavax HZ vaccine was reported to reduce the overall incidence of PHN by 39% (95% confidence interval [CI]: 7%–59%) in people 60 years of age and older who had developed zoster postvaccination and was shown to have the highest degree of effectiveness in subjects aged 70 to 79 years, whereby it reduced the incidence of PHN by 55% (95% CI: 18%–76%).[23]

The effectiveness of lessening the risk for PHN by reducing the overall severity of the acute phase of HZ through the use of antiviral drugs (eg, acyclovir, famciclovir, or valacyclovir) initiated within the first 72 hours after the HZ rash onset and continued for 7 days remains controversial because of conflicting evidence in the literature. Some studies suggest that antiviral drugs used in this manner for HZ significantly reduce the incidence of PHN, whereas others report no significant reduction in PHN incidence.[47,48]

Amitriptyline, corticosteroids, and gabapentin have each been advocated to help prevent the development of PHN when administered during acute HZ in a manner similar to that previously described for antiviral drugs.[27] However, it seems that only amitriptyline has shown a mild beneficial effect in the prevention of PHN in randomized controlled trials.[49]

Once PHN develops, its pharmacologic treatment follows the same general principle as seen with other types of chronic neuropathic pain and cranial neuralgias. Because the pathophysiology of PHN involves multiple, distinct processes within the peripheral nervous system and the CNS, the basis for pharmacologic treatment of PHN frequently involves the concurrent use of 2 or more drugs with different, complementary mechanisms of action that are designed to target multiple sites along the PHN pain pathways and interrupt the development, persistence, and perception of PHN.[43,50] However, the mechanisms by which different pharmacotherapies relieve PHN pain are not clearly understood.

First-line drugs used in the treatment of PHN typically include tricyclic antidepressants (eg, amitriptyline, desipramine, nortriptyline), gabapentinoids (eg, gabapentin, pregabalin), and topical lidocaine 5% patch. Opioid analgesics (eg, controlled release oxycodone, extended release morphine), nonopioid centrally acting analgesics (eg, tramadol, tapentadol), capsaicin 0.075% cream, and capsaicin 8% patch are typically recommended as either second- or third-line therapies in different PHN treatment guidelines.[43] Further information concerning pharmacotherapy for PHN is beyond the scope of this article, and the reader may wish to consult the cited references.[42,48,51,52]

REFERENCES

1. Okeson JP. Neuropathic pain. In: Bell's orofacial pains: the clinical management of orofacial pain. 6th edition. Chicago: Quintessence; 2005. p. 449–517.
2. Aguggia M. Typical facial neuralgias. Neurol Sci 2005;26(Suppl 2):s68–70.
3. De Simone R, Ranieri A, Bilo L, et al. Cranial neuralgias: from physiopathology to pharmacological treatment. Neurol Sci 2008;29(Suppl 1):S69–78.
4. Teixeira MJ, de Siqueira SR, Bor-Seng-Shu E. Glossopharyngeal neuralgia: neurosurgical treatment and differential diagnosis. Acta Neurochir (Wien) 2008;150(5):471–5 [discussion: 475].
5. Headache Classification Committee of the International Headache Society. Classification and diagnostic criteria for headache disorders, cranial neuralgias and facial pain. Cephalgia 2004;24(Suppl 1):122–36.
6. Obermann M, Katsarava Z. Update on trigeminal neuralgia. Expert Rev Neurother 2009;9(3):323–9.
7. Lewis MO, Sankar V, De Laat A, et al. Management of neuropathic orofacial pain. Oral Surg Oral Med Oral Pathol Oral Radiol Endod 2007;103(Suppl): S32.e1–24.
8. Benoliel R, Eliav E. Neuropathic orofacial pain. Oral Maxillofac Surg Clin North Am 2008;20(2):237–54, vii.
9. Spencer CJ, Gremillion HA. Neuropathic orofacial pain: proposed mechanisms, diagnosis, and treatment considerations. Dent Clin North Am 2007;51(1): 209–24, viii.

10. Zakrzewska JM. Medical management of trigeminal neuropathic pains. Expert Opin Pharmacother 2010;11(8):1239–54.
11. Stanic S, Franklin SD, Pappas CT, et al. Gamma knife radiosurgery for recurrent glossopharyngeal neuralgia after microvascular decompression. Stereotact Funct Neurosurg 2012;90(3):188–91.
12. Kawasaki M, Hatashima S, Matsuda T. Non-surgical therapy for bilateral glosso-pharyngeal neuralgia caused by Eagle's syndrome, diagnosed by three-dimensional computed tomography: a case report. J Anesth 2012;26(6):918–21.
13. Bruyn GW. Superior laryngeal neuralgia. Cephalalgia 1983;3(4):235–40.
14. Vanelderen P, Lataster A, Levy R, et al. Occipital neuralgia. Pain Pract 2010; 10(2):137–44.
15. Sulfaro MA, Gobetti JP. Occipital neuralgia manifesting as orofacial pain. Oral Surg Oral Med Oral Pathol Oral Radiol Endod 1995;80(6):751–5.
16. Shakur SF, Bhansali A, Mian AY, et al. Neurosurgical treatment of trigeminal neu-ralgia. Dis Mon 2011;57(10):570–82.
17. Larsen A, Piepgras D, Chyatte D, et al. Trigeminal neuralgia: diagnosis and medical and surgical management. JAAPA 2011;24(7):20–5.
18. Rozen TD. Trigeminal neuralgia and glossopharyngeal neuralgia. Neurol Clin 2004;22(1):185–206.
19. Zakrzewska JM, Akram H. Neurosurgical interventions for the treatment of clas-sical trigeminal neuralgia. Cochrane Database Syst Rev 2011;(9):CD007312.
20. Sampathkumar P, Drage LA, Martin DP. Herpes zoster (shingles) and posther-petic neuralgia. Mayo Clin Proc 2009;84(3):274–80.
21. Fashner J, Bell AL. Herpes zoster and postherpetic neuralgia: prevention and management. Am Fam Physician 2011;83(12):1432–7.
22. Johnson RW, Wasner G, Saddier P, et al. Postherpetic neuralgia: epidemiology, pathophysiology and management. Expert Rev Neurother 2007;7(11):1581–95.
23. Oxman MN, Levin MJ, Johnson GR, et al, Shingles Prevention Study Group. A vaccine to prevent herpes zoster and postherpetic neuralgia in older adults. N Engl J Med 2005;352:2271–84.
24. Weaver BA. The burden of herpes zoster and postherpetic neuralgia in the United States. J Am Osteopath Assoc 2007;107(Suppl 1):S2–7.
25. Jung BF, Johnson RW, Griffin DR, et al. Risk factors for postherpetic neuralgia in patients with herpes zoster. Neurology 2004;62(9):1545–51.
26. Johnson RW. Herpes zoster and postherpetic neuralgia. Expert Rev Vaccines 2010;9(Suppl 3):21–6.
27. Nalamachu S, Morley-Forster P. Diagnosing and managing postherpetic neural-gia. Drugs Aging 2012;29(11):863–9.
28. Kost RG, Straus SE. Postherpetic neuralgia–pathogenesis, treatment, and pre-vention. N Engl J Med 1996;335(1):32–42.
29. Philip A, Thakur R. Post herpetic neuralgia. J Palliat Med 2011;14(6):765–73.
30. Liesegang TJ. Herpes zoster ophthalmicus natural history, risk factors, clinical presentation, and morbidity. Ophthalmology 2008;115(Suppl 2):S3–12.
31. Sanjay S, Huang P, Lavanya R. Herpes zoster ophthalmicus. Curr Treat Options Neurol 2011;13(1):79–91.
32. Garza I, Swanson JW, Cheshire WP, et al. Headache and other craniofacial pain. In: Daroff RD, Fenichel GM, Jankovic J, et al, editors. Bradley's neurology in clin-ical practice. 6th edition. Philadelphia: Elsevier Saunders; 2012. Chapter 69. p. 1703–44.
33. Kim D, Bhimani M. Ramsay Hunt syndrome presenting as simple otitis externa. CJEM 2008;10(3):247–50.

34. Ragozzino MW, Melton LJ III, Kurland LT, et al. Population-based study of herpes zoster and its sequelae. Medicine (Baltimore) 1982;61:310–6.
35. Yawn BP, Saddier P, Wollan P, et al. A population-based study of the incidence and complication rates of herpes zoster before zoster vaccine introduction. Mayo Clin Proc 2007;82(11):1341–9 [published correction appears in Mayo Clin Proc 2008;83(2):255].
36. Zaal MJ, Völker-Diebe HJ, D'Amaro J. Risk and prognostic factors of postherpetic neuralgia and focal sensory denervation: a prospective evaluation in acute herpes zoster ophthalmicus. Clin J Pain 2000;16:345–51.
37. Scott FT, Leedham-Green ME, Barrett-Muir WY, et al. A study of shingles and the development of postherpetic neuralgia in East London. J Med Virol 2003;70: S24–30.
38. Higa K, Mori M, Hirata K, et al. Severity of skin lesions of herpes zoster at the worst phase rather than age and involved region most influences the duration of acute herpetic pain. Pain 1997;69:245–53.
39. Herr H. Prognostic factors of postherpetic neuralgia. J Korean Med Sci 2002;17: 655–9.
40. High KP. Preventing herpes zoster and postherpetic neuralgia through vaccination. J Fam Pract 2007;56(10 Suppl A):51A–7A.
41. Bowsher D. Pathophysiology of postherpetic neuralgia: towards a rational treatment. Neurology 1995;45(12 Suppl 8):S56–7.
42. Thakur R, Philip AG. Chronic pain perspectives: treating herpes zoster and postherpetic neuralgia: an evidence-based approach. J Fam Pract 2012; 61(Suppl 9):S9–15.
43. Argoff CE. Review of current guidelines on the care of postherpetic neuralgia. Postgrad Med 2011;123(5):134–42.
44. Truini A, Galeotti F, Haanpaa M, et al. Pathophysiology of pain in postherpetic neuralgia: a clinical and neurophysiological study. Pain 2008;140(3):405–10.
45. Schmader K. Herpes zoster in the elderly issues related to geriatrics. Clin Infect Dis 1999;28:736–9.
46. Dworkin RH, Portenoy RK. Pain and its persistence in herpes zoster. Pain 1996; 67:241–51.
47. Li Q, Chen N, Yang J, et al. Antiviral treatment for preventing postherpetic neuralgia. Cochrane Database Syst Rev 2009;(2):CD006866.
48. Watson PN. Postherpetic neuralgia. Clin Evid (Online) 2010. Available at: http:// clinicalevidence.bmj.com/ceweb/conditions/ind/0905/0905.jsp. Accessed January 28, 2013.
49. Bowsher D. The effects of pre-emptive treatment of post herpetic neuralgia with amitriptyline: a randomized, double- blind, placebo-controlled trial. J Pain Symptom Manage 1997;13:327.
50. Dworkin RH, O'Connor AB, Backonja M, et al. Pharmacologic management of neuropathic pain: evidence-based recommendations. Pain 2007;132(3): 237–51.
51. Whitley RJ, Volpi A, McKendrick M, et al. Management of herpes zoster and post-herpetic neuralgia now and in the future. J Clin Virol 2010;48(Suppl 1): S20–8.
52. Edelsberg JS, Lord C, Oster G. Systematic review and meta-analysis of efficacy, safety, and tolerability data from randomized controlled trials of drugs used to treat postherpetic neuralgia. Ann Pharmacother 2011;45(12):1483–90.

Burning Mouth Syndrome

Jaisri R. Thoppay, BDS, MBA[a], Scott S. De Rossi, DMD[b,c,d],
Katharine N. Ciarrocca, DMD, MSEd[d,e],*

KEYWORDS

- Burning mouth syndrome • Oral burning • Glossodynia • Oral dysesthesia

KEY POINTS

- The symptoms associated with burning mouth syndrome (BMS) can be quite varied and can have a negative impact on oral health-related quality of life.
- Management of BMS can be challenging for clinicians, because the treatment is aimed at the relief of symptoms without a definitive cure.
- Most randomized clinical trials on BMS treatment are inconclusive. Further investigations with larger patient populations and longer duration of treatment and follow-up are necessary to determine the true efficacy of different therapies. This is the only way viable therapeutic options for patients who suffer from this chronic and painful syndrome can be established.

INTRODUCTION
Disease Description

Burning mouth syndrome (BMS) afflicts more than one million adults in the US population, primarily affecting postmenopausal women between the ages of 50 to 70 years. Patients present complaining of oral burning and, because of the wide array of potential clinical factors, the diagnosis of this condition and treatment remain poorly understood.[1,2]

Risk Factors

- Gastrointestinal and urogenital problems were identified as risk factors that were solely associated with BMS.[3]
- Patients with BMS were characterized as having mild sensory and autonomic small-fiber neuropathy with concomitant central disorders.[4]

[a] College of Graduate Studies, Georgia Regents University, 1430 John Wesley Gilbert Drive, Augusta, GA 3091, USA; [b] Department of Otolaryngology/Head & Neck Surgery, Medical College of Georgia, Georgia Regents University, 1120 15th Street, Augusta, GA 30912, USA; [c] Department of Dermatology, Medical College of Georgia, Georgia Regents University, 1120 15th Street, Augusta, GA 30912, USA; [d] Division of Geriatric Dentistry, Department of Oral Health & Diagnostic Sciences, Georgia Regents University, College of Dental Medicine, 1430 John Wesley Gilbert Drive, GC4336, Augusta, GA 30912, USA; [e] Department of Oral Rehabilitation, Georgia Regents University, College of Dental Medicine, 1430 John Wesley Gilbert Drive, GC4336, Augusta, GA 30912, USA
* Corresponding author.
E-mail address: kciarrocca@gerogiahealth.edu

Dent Clin N Am 57 (2013) 497–512
http://dx.doi.org/10.1016/j.cden.2013.04.010
0011-8532/13/$ – see front matter © 2013 Published by Elsevier Inc.

- Medication (eg, angiotensin-converting enzyme inhibitors,[5] hypotensives, and diuretics) induced BMS[6]
- BMS after cessation of smoking[4]

Prevalence/Incidence

The prevalence of BMS has been reported to affect a wide range of the population. One study reported a prevalence from 0.7% to 5%[7,8] of the general population, and other studies reported between 3.7%[9] and 18% and even up to 40%.[10] One commonality among the studies is that BMS predominantly affects older age groups, especially postmenopausal women.[11,12] The reason that there is a wide range of reported prevalence figures of BMS is multifactorial. First, many published studies do not distinguish between the symptom of oral burning and the syndrome itself. Second, there is lack of consistency in the definition of the disease. Finally, there is variation in the study methodology, such as survey versus clinical assessment and geographic location.[2,7,12–14] The result is that the true prevalence of BMS is difficult to establish (**Table 1**).

CLINICAL CORRELATION
Introduction

Nature of problem
BMS is a complex disorder of unclear cause with the patient presenting with oral mucosal burning, which may be accompanied with xerostomia and dysguesia.

- The complexity of presenting symptoms and signs show difficulty for the patient and the practitioner evaluating these individuals in attaining the diagnosis.
- There are many factors that can contribute to the presenting symptoms.
- An evidence-based criteria derived from reliable and consistent scientific data will eliminate the difficulty in establishing a sound classification system for BMS.[19–21]

Definition
BMS is defined as a burning painful sensation in the mouth (oral dysesthesia) with normal clinical examination and no obvious organic cause. BMS is therefore a diagnosis of exclusion, made only after excluding all other causes of mouth pain. Evidence suggests that this disorder has a multifactorial cause, with neurologic, psychogenic, and hormonal factors all contributing to the disease.[10,22] Many names have been given to this condition, including orodynia (burning mouth) and glossodynia (burning tongue) being the 2 most common.

Symptoms
Oral pain is the major symptom and is most commonly described as a burning sensation like a scald from a hot drink, or as tingling or numbness. The tongue is the most common site involved, followed by the inside of the lower lip, and the hard palate (**Table 2**).

Table 1 Prevalence/incidence	
Age	• Commonly reported in women between the ages of 50s and 70s[13,15,16] • Rare under the age of 30[9,17]
Gender	• Female:male range from 3:1 to 16:1[18] • Present 3 y before and 12 y after menopause age[9,13] in women

Table 2 Symptoms	
Symptoms—Sensory, Chemosensory Abnormalities	

Persistent or constant oral mucosal pain daily[13]	• Burning, scalding, numb feeling, tingling
	  ○ Location (one or more)—tongue, oral mucosa, oropharyngeal areas, lips, nasal mucosa
	  ○ Intensity—variable, weak to intense
	  ○ Pattern/timing—continuous, not paroxysmal
	  ○ Localization—often bilateral, symmetric, independent of nervous pathways.
	Types:
	Three patterns of oral pain have been identified[23]:
	    Type 1: pain absent on waking and developing during the day
	    Type 2: pain present day and night
	    Type 3: intermittent pain, with pain-free days

Dysguesia 70%[13,24,25]	Persistent taste, altered taste, metallic taste, bitter taste[11]
Xerostomia 46%–67%[9,26]	With or without salivary gland hypofunction

Clinical Findings

Examination

A thorough history is vital in arriving at a definitive diagnosis and should include a present illness with previous treatments listed, a detailed past medical history, a complete list of current medications, and a thorough review of systems. An exhaustive extra-oral and intraoral examination should be performed following a detailed history. Local factors, such as denture fit and design, dental trauma, signs of parafunctional habits, mechanical or chemical irritant, infection, hyposalivation, lesions, and allergies,[27] should be the focus.

Diagnostic Modalities

The diagnosis of BMS is often complex due to the following multiple reasons:

- The diagnosis relies on the patient's presenting symptoms
- The symptomatic triad is rarely present or overlapping of other contributing factors
- The diagnosis is obtained after eliminating other potential causes for oral burning.

Symptomatically, BMS must be differentiated from other chronic oral pain conditions. A careful evaluation of any structure in the head and neck complex that may potentially cause oral pain should be performed. In addition, further evaluation is needed to rule out underlying etiologic factors from a systemic factor (**Fig. 1**).

The following additional evaluations may be necessary:

- Sialometry to evaluate the oral dryness[13]
  - Unstimulated whole saliva ≥ 0.1 mg/min
  - Stimulated whole saliva ≥ 0.7 mg/min
- Biopsy of minor salivary glands if Sjogren syndrome is suspected
- Biopsy or cytology if any oral mucosal lesions will be included in differential diagnosis[18,28]
- Culture of oral samples, to rule out fungal, viral, and bacterial infections

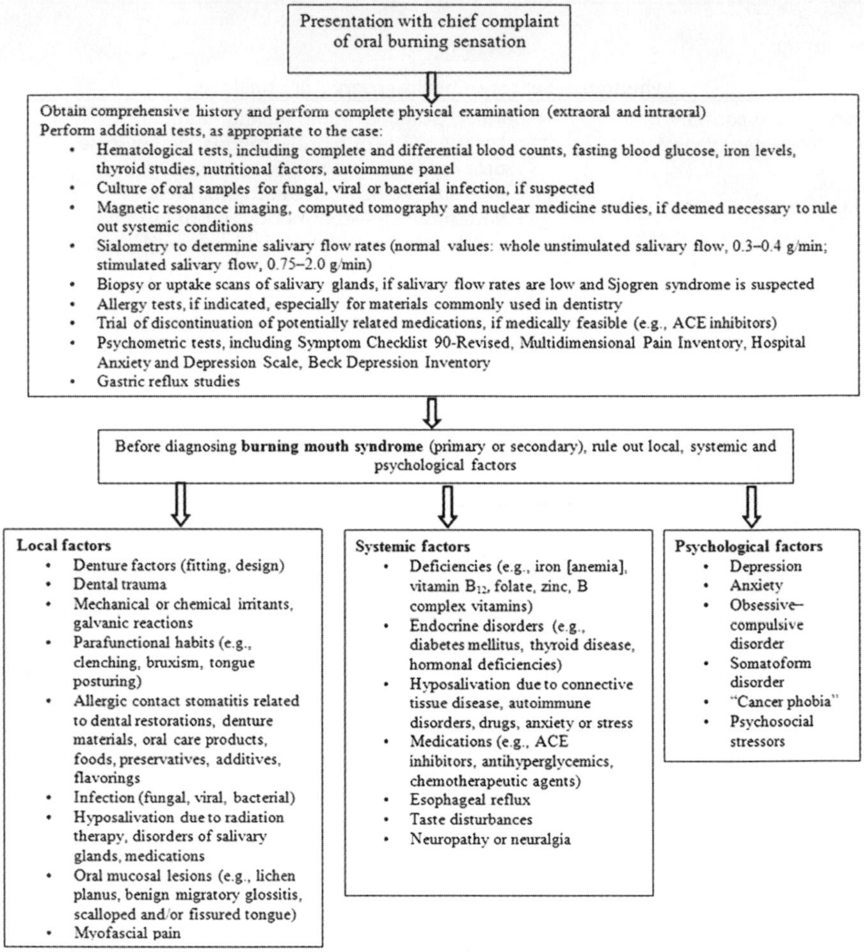

Fig. 1. Algorithm for diagnostic considerations in patients with oral burning sensation. ACE, angiotensin-converting enzyme. (*From* Klasser G, Epstein J, Villines D. Diagnostic dilemma: the enigma of an oral burning sensation. J Can Dent Assoc 2011;77:b146; with permission.)

- Hematological test that may include complete and differential blood counts, fasting blood sugar levels, thyroid panel, nutritional factors (to rule out deficiencies such as iron, folate, and B12), autoimmune panel (ANA, Rf, Anti-SSA, Anti-SSB)
- Skin patch test to rule out any allergic reaction[29]
- Magnetic resonance imaging if BMS is associated with neuralgia or trigeminal nerve neuropathy is included in differential and to rule out systemic conditions
- Trial of discontinuation of medications, such as angiotensin-converting enzyme inhibitors,[5] known to cause symptoms may be considered
- Psychometric tests, including symptoms Checklist 90 revised, multidimensional pain inventory, hospital anxiety and depression scale, Beck Depression Inventory, can be considered to evaluate the influence of psychological factors[30,31]
- Gastric reflex studies may also be considered.

Pathologic Condition

The pathophysiology of BMS is complex. Evidence from multiple studies suggests hormonal,[32–34] neuropathic,[16,35] and psychological,[22,30,37] all as potential etiologic factors

- Hormone balance may be related to BMS in women, because the disease is more frequent during and after menopause, but clinical studies yielded controversial results with hormone replacement therapies[32,33]
- Neuropathic causes: 3 distinct subclasses have been classified[10,16,38]:
  - Peripheral small-fiber neuropathy
  - Subclinical major trigeminal neuropathy
  - Central pain that may be related to deficient dopaminergic top-down inhibition.
- Psychological profile showing personality and mood changes.[4,39–41]

Diagnostic Dilemmas

Historically, BMS has been referred to by many names and defined depending on location and associated conditions in over 300 published articles for the past 10 years. These definitions and classification show difficulty for the patient and the practitioner evaluating these individuals in attaining the diagnosis. However, the current classification is based on various diagnostic criteria based on symptoms and causes (**Table 3**).

Comorbidities

Evidence suggests a wide range of comorbid conditions associated with BMS.

- Systemic conditions
  - Psychiatric disorders
  - Diabetes
  - Gastroenteric diseases
- Local conditions
  - Benign migratory glossitis
  - Oral lichen planus
  - Xerostomia
  - Taste disturbances
  - Candidiasis
  - Trigeminal neuralgia

Case studies

- BMS has high psychiatric comorbidity but can occur in the absence of psychiatric diagnoses[36,37,45]
- Oral lichen planus
- BMS and peripheral neuropathy in patients with type 1 diabetes mellitus[46,47]
- Increased prevalence of benign migratory glossitis with BMS[28]
- *Helicobacter pylori* colonization of tongue mucosa—increased incidence in atrophic glossitis and BMS[48]
- Glossodynia from Candida-associated lesions, BMS, or mixed causes[49–51]
- Pain intensity and psychosocial characteristics of patients with BMS and trigeminal neuralgia[52,53]
- BMS and xerostomia[54]

Table 3
Classification of BMS

Source, Year	Diagnostic Criteria
Fortuna et al,[42] 2013	Suggests rename as complex oral sensitivity disorder (COSD) and defines as an oropharyngeal discomfort due to one or more symptoms for which no specific cause of any type can be identified in the following criteria 1. Any type of oropharyngeal symptom that can be persistent or intermittent with possible phases of remission/exacerbation during the day; 2. Absence of any clinically and instrumentally detectable oropharyngeal lesion; 3. Absence of any type of local and/or systemic factors such as oral diseases, drugs, trauma, hypersensitivity reactions, physical/chemical agents.
ICHD II, 2004[43]	Describes as an intra-oral burning sensation for which no medical or dental cause can be found and the diagnostic criteria as follows: A. Pain in the mouth present daily and presenting most of the day B. Oral mucosa is of normal appearance C. Local and systemic diseases have been excluded. Comment: Pain may be confined to the tongue (glossodynia) with or without xerostomia, paresthesia, and dysgeusia
Scala et al,[2] 2003	1. Primary BMS or essential/idiopathic BMS with no organic or systemic cause 2. Secondary BMS resulting from local/systemic cause.

Muzyka & De Rossi,[1] 1999	**Type Percentage Symptoms**
	1 35% • Awaken without symptoms
	          • Progress throughout the day
	          • Present daily
	          • Food/drink relieve symptoms
	2 55% • Awaken with symptoms
	          • Progress daily
	          • Food/drink relieve symptoms
	3 10% • Occasional symptoms
	          • Worsen with food/drink
	          • Unusual oral sites affected
	          • Increases incidence of contact allergy

International Association for the Study of Pain (IASP) (Merksey and Bogduk), 1994[44]	Defined as "all forms of burning sensation in the mouth, including complaints described as stinging sensation or pain, in association with an oral mucosa that appears clinically normal in the absence of local or systemic diseases or alterations"
Lamey & Lewis,[23] 1989	Type 1: progressive pain throughout the day Type 2: constant throughout the day Type 3: symptoms are intermittent and there are some symptom-free days

Management

BMS is a challenging condition in terms of both diagnosis and management. Intervention is often undertaken while working on establishing a definitive diagnosis.[19,55] The process of eliminating the underlying cause is stepwise and often time-consuming, which prompts the initiation of empiric treatment toward the presenting clinical signs and symptoms.

Challenges in management strategies include the following:

- Despite the existence of evidence-based management approaches, there is usually a delay in establishing a definitive diagnosis from the onset of symptoms, which ranges from 1 to 34 months with an average of 13 months.[21]
- The average number of medical and dental practitioners consulted by each patient over this period and who initially misdiagnosed BMS was 3.1 (range, 0 to 12; median, 3). Oral burning due to Candidiasis and aspecific stomatitis were the most frequent misinterpretations of the symptoms before appropriate referral. In about 30% of the cases, no diagnosis of the oral symptoms was made or explanation given.[21]
- It is evident from many studies that the complexity of diagnostic enigma had been a challenge to distinguish between burning complains and true syndrome for practitioners.[19,22]

Goals

Management strategies for effective outcome include the following:

- Establishing a definitive diagnosis—separating oral burning from BMS, ruling out local and systemic causes of oral burning that is not pertinent to definitive diagnosis of BMS.[8,18,19]
- Understanding the local, systemic, and psychological factors that may be responsible for oral burning associated with secondary BMS and therefore a foundation for diagnosing primary BMS.[18,19,56]
- Establishing a treatment plan based on the presenting symptoms and clinical presentations in the initial visit and treatment modifications based on investigations and prior treatment outcomes in the following visits.

Pharmacologic strategies

BMS is a multifactorial chronic neuropathic condition that requires therapeutic strategies that include pharmacologic interventions directly relating to the symptoms and/or treating the underlying local, systemic, and/or psychological factors. These strategies target different factors that may be directly related to the symptoms and signs or to the subclinical neuropathic condition.[8,55]

Treatment strategy can be based on the following:

- Palliative
- Symptomatic
- Therapeutic
- Combinations of the above

Patient education on this syndrome is vital, and patients need to be informed about the characteristics of the condition and to be aware of the existing therapeutic difficulties and true possibilities of symptom relief. However, management is multidisciplinary,[57] often necessitating modification of the treatment plan until a stable effective management protocol is achieved. Depending on the outcome, the patient management protocol can be modified or tapered until resolved. The management approaches suggested[57] in the literature are follows:

Step 1: Diagnose and manage local and systemic cofactors related to secondary BMS

- Local
  - Oral examination
  - Salivary hypofunction/xerostomia
  - Parafunctional habits
  - Contact allergies
- Systemic
  - Hematological parameters
  - Nutritional deficiencies
  - Hormonal disturbances
  - Side effects from medications
- Psychological factors

Step 2: Multidisciplinary management of primary or idiopathic BMS

Based on published randomized clinical trials:

- Topical
  - Clonazepam[58]
- Systemic
  - α-Lipoic acid[59]
  - Selective serotonin reuptake inhibitors (paroxetine,[60] sertraline)
  - Amisulpride[61,62]
  - Anticonvulsants (gabapentin)[63]
- Cognitive behavioral therapy[64]

Based on expert opinion and common clinical practice but not yet evaluated

- Topical
  - Capsaicin
  - Doxepin
  - Lidocaine
- Systemic
  - Tricyclic antidepressants
  - Serotonin-norepinephrine reuptake inhibitors
  - Anticonvulsants
  - Opioids
  - Benzodiazepines—Clonazepam, Alprazolam

Topical medications Table 4 lists the topical medications for BMS.

Systemic medication Table 5 lists the systemic medications for BMS.

Nonpharmacologic strategies
Nonpharmacologic treatment modalities should include the following:

- Cessation of parafunctional habits, such as clenching, bruxism, tongue protrusion, that may contribute to oral burning. Desensitizing appliances can be used to reduce oral burning and can also be used as a habit-breaking appliance.[67]
- Modification of oral care products, such as alcohol-free mouthwashes, and regular oral care products without flavoring agents can be considered
- Patients with influence of psychological factors could be counseled for stress management.[30,31]

Evaluation of outcome and long-term recommendations
Therapeutic outcomes Table 6 lists the therapeutic outcomes of BMS.

Clinical outcomes Table 7 lists the clinical outcomes for BMS.

Complications and concerns Table 8 lists the complications and concerns for BMS.

Table 4
Topical medications

Medications	Specific Examples	Dose	Directions
Benzodiazepines	Klonazepam wafer/orally disintegrating tablets[58]	0.25 mg–2 mg/d	0.25 mg at bedtime; increase dosage by 0.25 mg every 4 to 7 d until oral burning is relieved or side effects occur; as dosage increases, medication is taken as full dose or in 3 divided doses
Anesthetic	Lidocaine 2% viscous gel	Variable	Applied PRN on the oral mucoca/tongue
Atypical analgesic	Capsacin cream	Variable	Rinse mouth with 1 teaspoon of a 1:2 dilution (or higher) of hot pepper and water; increase strength of capsaicin as tolerated to a maximum of 1:1 dilution.
Anti-depressant	Doxepin 5% cream	Variable	Q4–6 h
Nonsteroidal anti-inflammatory	Benzydamine oral rinse	Variable	Dispense 5 mL, swish for 30 s, and spit, TID
Antimicrobial	Lactoperoxidase oral rinse	Variable	Dispense 5 mL, swish for 30 s, and spit, BID
Mucosal protectant	Sucralfate oral rinse	Variable	Dispense 5 mL, swish for 30 s, and spit, TID

Table 5
Systemic medications

Medications	Specific Examples	Dose	Directions
Benzodiazepine (low dose)	Clonazepam	0.5–2 mg/d	0.25 mg at bedtime; increase dosage by 0.25 mg every 4 to 7 d until oral burning is relieved or side effects occur; as dosage increases, medication is taken as full dose or in 3 divided doses
	Chlordiazepoxide	10–30 mg/d	5 mg at bedtime; increase dosage by 5 mg every 4 to 7 d until oral burning is relieved or side effects occur; as dosage increases, medication is taken in 3 divided doses
Anticonvulsants	Gabapentin	300 to 1600 mg/d	100 mg at bedtime; increase dosage by 100 mg every 4 to 7 d until oral burning is relieved or side effects occur; as dosage increases, medication is taken in 3 divided doses
	Pregabalin	25 to 300 mg	25 mg at bedtime; increase dosage by 25 mg every 4 to 7 d until oral burning is relieved or side effects occur; as dosage increases, medication is taken in 3 divided doses
Antidepressants (low dose)	Amitriptyline	10 to 150 mg/d	10 mg at bedtime; increase dosage by 10 mg every 4 to 7 d until oral burning is relieved or side effects occur
	Nortriptyline	10 to 150 mg/d	10 mg at bedtime; increase dosage by 10 mg every 4 to 7 d until oral burning is relieved or side effects occur
Selective serotonin reuptake inhibitors	Paroxetine	20–50 mg/d	10 to 150 mg QAM
	Sertraline	50–200 mg/d	Start 50 mg PO QD, may increase 25–50 mg every 4 to 7 d until oral burning is relieved or side effects occur, max. 200 mg/d
	Trazodone	100 mg–400 mg/d	Start 50 mg PO BID/TID, may increase 50 mg every 4 to 7 d until oral burning is relieved or side effects occur, max. 400 mg/d

(continued on next page)

Table 5
(continued)

Medications	Specific Examples	Dose	Directions
Selective norepinephrine reuptake inhibitors	Milnacipran	100 mg/d	50 mg BID, start with 12.5 mg, then 12.5 BID every 4 to 7 d until oral burning is relieved or side effects occur, max. 200 mg/d
	Duloxetine[65,66]	60 mg–120 mg/d	60 mg–120 mg PO QD
Antioxidant	α-Lipoic acid	600 mg–1200 mg	300 mg/600 mg BID
Atypical antipsychotic	Olanzipine	5–20 mg/d	5–20 mg PO QPM
Dopamine agonist	Pramipexole	0.125–0.5 mg PO QPM	Start 0.125 mg PO QPM, may increase 0.125 mg/d q4–7 d max. 0.5 mg/d, 2–3 h before bedtime
Herbal supplement	Hypericum perforatum (St John's wort)	300 mg to 1800 mg/d in divided doses	300 mg TID
Salivary stimulants	Pilocarpaine Cevimiline	15–40 mg/d 90–120 mg/d	5 mg/10 mg TID/QID 30 mg TID/QID

Table 6
Therapeutic outcomes

Author, Year	Study	Outcome
Amos et al,[68] 2011	Combined topical and systemic clonazepam therapy for the management of burning mouth syndrome	Combined topical and systemic clonazepam administration provides an effective BMS management tool
Silvestre-Rangil et al,[69] 2011	Correlation of treatment to clinical variables of the disease	The greatest treatment efficacy corresponded to anxiolytic drugs, and treatment was more effective when introduced early after the diagnosis of BMS
Barker et al,[70] 2009	Comparison of treatment modalities in burning mouth syndrome	Patients taking clonazepam reported either partial or complete relief of symptoms compared with diazepam
Steele et al,[71] 2008	α-Lipoic acid treatment of 31 patients with sore, burning mouth	Patients (35%) reported benefit from taking α-lipoic acid

Table 7		
Clinical outcomes		
Author, Year	**Study**	**Outcome**
Ching et al,[28] 2012	Increased prevalence of benign migratory glossitis (BMG) in BMS patients	Prevalence = 26.7% in the study group, suggesting BMG may be a significant predictor for BMS
Rouleau et al,[72] 2011	The prevalence and risk factors of oral burning in patients with dry mouth	Oral burning is often concomitant with oral dryness
Femiano et al,[73] 2008	Burning mouth disorder (BMD) and taste: a hypothesis	BMD may represent an oral phantom pain induced in susceptible individuals by alteration of taste
Sardella et al,[74] 2006	A retrospective study investigating spontaneous remission and response to treatments	Complete spontaneous remission was observed in 3% of the patients within 5 y after the onset of BMS. A moderate improvement was obtained in <30% of the subjects
Pinto et al,[75] 2003	A retrospective analysis of clinical characteristics and treatment outcomes	No significant correlation between classification of BMS and response to therapy. The most effective treatment modalities were habit awareness, followed by TCAs

Table 8		
Complications and concerns		
Author, Year	**Study**	**Outcome**
Klasser et al,[76] 2011	Challenge for dental practitioners and patients	Patients frequently reported delays in receiving a definitive diagnosis with an array of various trialed interventions
Mignogna et al,[21] 2005	The diagnosis of burning mouth syndrome represents a challenge for clinicians	The average number of medical and dental practitioners consulted by each patient over this period and who initially misdiagnosed BMS was 3.1 (range, 0 to 12; median, 3). Candidiasis and aspecific stomatitis were the most frequent misinterpretations of the symptoms before appropriate referral. In about 30% of cases, no diagnosis of the oral symptoms was made or explanation given

SUMMARY

The symptoms associated with BMS can be quite varied and can have a negative impact on oral health-related quality of life.[77] Management of BMS can be challenging for clinicians, as the treatment is aimed at the relief of symptoms without a definitive cure. Most randomized clinical trials on BMS treatment are inconclusive. Further investigations with larger patient populations and longer duration of treatment and follow-up are necessary to determine the true efficacy of different therapies. This is the only way viable therapeutic options for patients who suffer from this chronic and painful syndrome[59] can be established.

REFERENCES

1. Muzyka BC, De Rossi SS. A review of burning mouth syndrome. Cutis 1999; 64(1):29–35.
2. Scala A, Checchi L, Montevecchi M, et al. Update on burning mouth syndrome: overview and patient management. Crit Rev Oral Biol Med 2003; 14(4):275–91.
3. Netto FO, Diniz IM, Grossmann SM, et al. Risk factors in burning mouth syndrome: a case-control study based on patient records. Clin Oral Investig 2011;15(4):571–5.
4. Gao J, Chen L, Zhou J, et al. A case-control study on etiological factors involved in patients with burning mouth syndrome. J Oral Pathol Med 2009;38(1):24–8.
5. Savino LB, Haushalter NM. Lisinopril-induced "scalded mouth syndrome". Ann Pharmacother 1992;26(11):1381–2.
6. Salort-Llorca C, Minguez-Serra MP, Silvestre FJ. Drug-induced burning mouth syndrome: a new etiological diagnosis. Med Oral Patol Oral Cir Bucal 2008; 13(3):E167–70.
7. Klausner J. Epidemiology of chronic facial pain: diagnostic usefulness in patient care. J Am Dent Assoc 1994;125(12):1604–11.
8. Klasser GD, Epstein JB. Oral burning and burning mouth syndrome. J Am Dent Assoc 2012;143(12):1317–9.
9. Bergdahl M, Bergdahl J. Burning mouth syndrome: prevalence and associated factors. J Oral Pathol Med 1999;28(8):350–4.
10. Jaaskelainen SK. Pathophysiology of primary burning mouth syndrome. Clin Neurophysiol 2012;123(1):71–7.
11. Ship JA, Grushka M, Lipton JA, et al. Burning mouth syndrome: an update. J Am Dent Assoc 1995;126(7):842–53.
12. Grushka M, Epstein JB, Gorsky M. Burning mouth syndrome. Am Fam Physician 2002;65(4):615–20.
13. Grushka M. Clinical features of burning mouth syndrome. Oral Surg Oral Med Oral Pathol 1987;63(1):30–6.
14. Eguia Del Valle A, Aguirre-Urizar JM, Martinez-Conde R, et al. Burning mouth syndrome in the Basque Country: a preliminary study of 30 cases. Med Oral 2003;8(2):84–90.
15. Zakrzewska JM. The burning mouth syndrome remains an enigma. Pain 1995; 62(3):253–7.
16. Lauria G, Majorana A, Borgna M, et al. Trigeminal small-fiber sensory neuropathy causes burning mouth syndrome. Pain 2005;115(3):332–7.
17. Danhauer SC, Miller CS, Rhodus NL, et al. Impact of criteria-based diagnosis of burning mouth syndrome on treatment outcome. J Orofac Pain 2002;16(4): 305–11.

18. Klasser GD, Epstein JB, Villines D. Diagnostic dilemma: the enigma of an oral burning sensation. J Can Dent Assoc 2011;77:b146.
19. Balasubramaniam R, Klasser GD, Delcanho R. Separating oral burning from burning mouth syndrome: unravelling a diagnostic enigma. Aust Dent J 2009; 54(4):293–9.
20. Mignogna MD, Pollio A, Fortuna G, et al. Unexplained somatic comorbidities in patients with burning mouth syndrome: a controlled clinical study. J Orofac Pain 2011;25(2):131–40.
21. Mignogna MD, Fedele S, Lo Russo L, et al. The diagnosis of burning mouth syndrome represents a challenge for clinicians. J Orofac Pain 2005;19(2):168–73.
22. Spanemberg JC, Cherubini K, de Figueiredo MA, et al. Aetiology and therapeutics of burning mouth syndrome: an update. Gerodontology 2012;29(2):84–9.
23. Lamey PJ, Lewis MA. Oral medicine in practice: burning mouth syndrome. Br Dent J 1989;167(6):197–200.
24. Grushka M, Sessle B. Taste dysfunction in burning mouth syndrome. Gerodontics 1988;4(5):256–8.
25. Main DM, Basker RM. Patients complaining of a burning mouth. Further experience in clinical assessment and management. Br Dent J 1983;154(7):206–11.
26. Gorsky M, Silverman S Jr, Chinn H. Burning mouth syndrome: a review of 98 cases. J Oral Med 1987;42(1):7–9.
27. Brown RS, Farquharson AA, Sam FE, et al. A retrospective evaluation of 56 patients with oral burning and limited clinical findings. Gen Dent 2006;54(4): 267–71.
28. Ching V, Grushka M, Darling M, et al. Increased prevalence of geographic tongue in burning mouth complaints: a retrospective study. Oral Surg Oral Med Oral Pathol Oral Radiol 2012;114(4):444–8.
29. Steele JC, Bruce AJ, Davis MD, et al. Clinically relevant patch test results in patients with burning mouth syndrome. Dermatitis 2012;23(2):61–70.
30. Abetz LM, Savage NW. Burning mouth syndrome and psychological disorders. Aust Dent J 2009;54(2):84–93.
31. Carlson CR, Miller CS, Reid KI. Psychosocial profiles of patients with burning mouth syndrome. J Orofac Pain 2000;14(1):59–64.
32. Tarkkila L, Linna M, Tiitinen A, et al. Oral symptoms at menopause–the role of hormone replacement therapy. Oral Surg Oral Med Oral Pathol Oral Radiol Endod 2001;92(3):276–80.
33. Forabosco A, Criscuolo M, Coukos G, et al. Efficacy of hormone replacement therapy in postmenopausal women with oral discomfort. Oral Surg Oral Med Oral Pathol 1992;73(5):570–4.
34. Wardrop RW, Hailes J, Burger H, et al. Oral discomfort at menopause. Oral Surg Oral Med Oral Pathol 1989;67(5):535–40.
35. Albuquerque RJ, de Leeuw R, Carlson CR, et al. Cerebral activation during thermal stimulation of patients who have burning mouth disorder: an fMRI study. Pain 2006;122(3):223–34.
36. Mendak-Ziolko M, Konopka T, Bogucki ZA. Evaluation of select neurophysiological, clinical and psychological tests for burning mouth syndrome. Oral Surg Oral Med Oral Pathol Oral Radiol 2012;114(3):325–32.
37. Kenchadze R, Iverieli M, Okribelashvili N, et al. The psychological aspects of burning mouth syndrome. Georgian Med News 2011;194:24–8.
38. Prakash S, Ahuja S, Rathod C. Dopa responsive burning mouth syndrome: restless mouth syndrome or oral variant of restless legs syndrome? J Neurol Sci 2012;320(1–2):156–60.

39. Femiano F, Gombos F, Scully C. Burning mouth syndrome: open trial of psycho-therapy alone, medication with alpha-lipoic acid (thioctic acid), and combination therapy. Med Oral 2004;9(1):8–13.
40. Shah B, Ashok L, Sujatha GP. Evaluation of salivary cortisol and psychological factors in patients with oral lichen planus. Indian J Dent Res 2009;20(3):288–92.
41. Schiavone V, Adamo D, Ventrella G, et al. Anxiety, depression, and pain in burning mouth syndrome: first chicken or egg? Headache 2012;52(6):1019–25.
42. Fortuna G, Lorenzo MD, Pollio A. Complex oral sensitivity disorder (COSD): a reappraisal of current classification of burning mouth syndrome. Oral Dis 2013. [Epub ahead of print].
43. International Headache Society. Available at: http://www.ihs-headache.org/. Accessed May 21, 2013.
44. International Association for the Sudy of Pain. Available at: www.iasp-pain.org/. Accessed May 21, 2013.
45. Bogetto F, Maina G, Ferro G, et al. Psychiatric comorbidity in patients with burning mouth syndrome. Psychosom Med 1998;60(3):378–85.
46. Moore PA, Guggenheimer J, Orchard T. Burning mouth syndrome and peripheral neuropathy in patients with type 1 diabetes mellitus. J Diabetes Complications 2007;21(6):397–402.
47. Moore PA, Zgibor JC, Dasanayake AP. Diabetes: a growing epidemic of all ages. J Am Dent Assoc 2003;134(Spec No):11S–5S.
48. Gall-Troselj K, Mravak-Stipetic M, Jurak I, et al. Helicobacter pylori colonization of tongue mucosa–increased incidence in atrophic glossitis and burning mouth syndrome (BMS). J Oral Pathol Med 2001;30(9):560–3.
49. Terai H, Shimahara M. Glossodynia from Candida-associated lesions, burning mouth syndrome, or mixed causes. Pain Med 2010;11(6):856–60.
50. Cavalcanti DR, Birman EG, Migliari DA, et al. Burning mouth syndrome: clinical profile of Brazilian patients and oral carriage of Candida species. Braz Dent J 2007;18(4):341–5.
51. Sardella A, Lodi G, Demarosi F, et al. Causative or precipitating aspects of burning mouth syndrome: a case-control study. J Oral Pathol Med 2006;35(8):466–71.
52. Komiyama O, Obara R, Uchida T, et al. Pain intensity and psychosocial characteristics of patients with burning mouth syndrome and trigeminal neuralgia. J Oral Sci 2012;54(4):321–7.
53. de Tommaso M, Lavolpe V, Di Venere D, et al. A case of unilateral burning mouth syndrome of neuropathic origin. Headache 2011;51(3):441–4.
54. da Silva LA, Teixeira MJ, de Siqueira JT, et al. Xerostomia and salivary flow in patients with orofacial pain compared with controls. Arch Oral Biol 2011; 56(10):1142–7.
55. Klasser GD, Epstein JB, Villines D. Management of burning mouth syndrome. J Mich Dent Assoc 2012;94(6):43–6.
56. Klasser GD, Epstein JB, Villines D. Management of burning mouth syndrome. J Can Dent Assoc 2011;77:b151.
57. Patton LL, Siegel MA, Benoliel R, et al. Management of burning mouth syndrome: systematic review and management recommendations. Oral Surg Oral Med Oral Pathol Oral Radiol 2007;103(Suppl):S39.e1–13.
58. Heckmann SM, Kirchner E, Grushka M, et al. A double-blind study on clonazepam in patients with burning mouth syndrome. Laryngoscope 2012;122(4):813–6.
59. de Moraes M, do Amaral Bezerra BA, da Rocha Neto PC, et al. Randomized trials for the treatment of burning mouth syndrome: an evidence-based review of the literature. J Oral Pathol Med 2012;41(4):281–7.

60. Yamazaki Y, Hata H, Kitamori S, et al. An open-label, noncomparative, dose escalation pilot study of the effect of paroxetine in treatment of burning mouth syndrome. Oral Surg Oral Med Oral Pathol Oral Radiol Endod 2009;107(1):8.

61. Rodriguez-Cerdeira C, Sanchez-Blanco E. Treatment of burning mouth syndrome with amisulpride. J Clin Med Res 2012;4(3):167–71.

62. Maina G, Vitalucci A, Gandolfo S, et al. Comparative efficacy of SSRIs and amisulpride in burning mouth syndrome: a single-blind study. J Clin Psychiatry 2002;63(1):38–43.

63. White TL, Kent PF, Kurtz DB, et al. Effectiveness of gabapentin for treatment of burning mouth syndrome. Arch Otolaryngol Head Neck Surg 2004;130(6): 786–8.

64. Van Houdenhove B, Joostens P. Burning mouth syndrome. Successful treatment with combined psychotherapy and psychopharmacotherapy. Gen Hosp Psychiatry 1995;17(5):385–8.

65. Nagashima W, Kimura H, Ito M, et al. Effectiveness of duloxetine for the treatment of chronic nonorganic orofacial pain. Clin Neuropharmacol 2012;35(6): 273–7.

66. Mignogna MD, Adamo D, Schiavone V, et al. Burning mouth syndrome responsive to duloxetine: a case report. Pain Med 2011;12(3):466–9.

67. Axell T. Treatment of smarting symptoms in the oral mucosa by appliance of lingual acrylic splints. Swed Dent J 2008;32(4):165–9.

68. Amos K, Yeoh SC, Farah CS. Combined topical and systemic clonazepam therapy for the management of burning mouth syndrome: a retrospective pilot study. J Orofac Pain 2011;25(2):125–30.

69. Silvestre-Rangil J, Silvestre FJ, Tamarit-Santafe C, et al. Burning mouth syndrome: correlation of treatment to clinical variables of the disease. Med Oral Patol Oral Cir Bucal 2011;16(7):e890–4.

70. Barker KE, Batstone MD, Savage NW. Comparison of treatment modalities in burning mouth syndrome. Aust Dent J 2009;54(4):300–5.

71. Steele JC, Bruce AJ, Drage LA, et al. Alpha-lipoic acid treatment of 31 patients with sore, burning mouth. Oral Dis 2008;14(6):529–32.

72. Rouleau TS, Shychuk AJ, Kayastha J, et al. A retrospective, cohort study of the prevalence and risk factors of oral burning in patients with dry mouth. Oral Surg Oral Med Oral Pathol Oral Radiol Endod 2011;111(6):720–5.

73. Femiano F, Lanza A, Buonaiuto C, et al. Burning mouth disorder (BMD) and taste: a hypothesis. Med Oral Patol Oral Cir Bucal 2008;13(8):E470–4.

74. Sardella A, Lodi G, Demarosi F, et al. Burning mouth syndrome: a retrospective study investigating spontaneous remission and response to treatments. Oral Dis 2006;12(2):152–5.

75. Pinto A, Sollecito TP, DeRossi SS. Burning mouth syndrome. A retrospective analysis of clinical characteristics and treatment outcomes. N Y State Dent J 2003;69(3):18–24.

76. Klasser GD, Epstein JB, Villines D, et al. Burning mouth syndrome: a challenge for dental practitioners and patients. Gen Dent 2011;59(3):210–20.

77. Ni Riordain R, Moloney E, O'Sullivan K, et al. Burning mouth syndrome and oral health-related quality of life: is there a change over time? Oral Dis 2010;16(7): 643–7.

Primary Headache Disorders

Rafael Benoliel, BDS, LDS RCS Eng[a],*, Eli Eliav, DMD, PhD[b]

KEYWORDS

- Migraine • Tension-type headaches • Trigeminal autonomic cephalgias
- Hemicrania continua

KEY POINTS

- Primary headache disorders include migraine, tension-type headaches, and the trigeminal autonomic cephalgias (TACs).
- "Primary" refers to a lack of clear underlying causative pathology, trauma, or systemic disease.
- The TACs include cluster headache (CH), paroxysmal hemicrania (PH), and short-lasting neuralgiform headache attacks with conjunctival injection and tearing (SUNCT); hemicrania continua (HC), although classified separately by the International Headache Society (IHS), shares many features with both migraine and the TACs.
- The IHS classification system is viewable at http://ihs-classification.org/en/.

INTRODUCTION

Primary headache disorders include migraine, tension-type headaches, and the trigeminal autonomic cephalgias (TACs). "Primary" refers to a lack of clear underlying causative pathology, trauma, or systemic disease.

The TACs include cluster headache (CH), paroxysmal hemicrania (PH), and short-lasting neuralgiform headache attacks with conjunctival injection and tearing (SUNCT); hemicrania continua (HC), although classified separately by the International Headache Society (IHS),[1] shares many features of both migraine and the TACs. The IHS classification system is viewable at http://ihs-classification.org/en/.

MIGRAINE

Migraine is a common primary headache with an additional number of rarer related syndromes.[1] Prevalence studies in Western countries show that migraine affects approximately 10% to 12% of the adult population, but figures are not always

[a] Department of Oral Medicine, The Faculty of Dentistry, Hebrew University-Hadassah, POB 12272, Jerusalem, Israel; [b] Division of Orofacial Pain, Department of Diagnostic Sciences, UMDNJ-New Jersey Dental School, 110 Bergen Street, Newark, NJ 07103, USA
* Corresponding author.
E-mail address: rafaelb@ekmd.huji.ac.il

Dent Clin N Am 57 (2013) 513–539
http://dx.doi.org/10.1016/j.cden.2013.04.005
0011-8532/13/$ – see front matter © 2013 Elsevier Inc. All rights reserved.

dental.theclinics.com

consistent.[2–5] The 2 most common types of migraine headaches are migraine without aura (MWA) and migraine with aura (MA).[6] The combination of a high prevalence, severe pain, and debilitating neurologic symptoms results in a substantial social impact with decreased quality of life.[7,8]

MWA is an inherited disorder affecting the young, with an onset before the age of 20 years in about half of the cases.[9] There is up to a twofold increase of MWA among first-degree relatives of patients with MWA and a fourfold increase in MA.[10,11] Studies suggest that multiple receptor polymorphisms and multigene inheritance are involved.[12,13]

Migraine presentation may be divided into phases and each may occur alone or in combination with each other. The headache phase is identical in MA and MWA.

- Prodrome
  - Premonitory signs and symptoms occurring days or hours before some or all headaches.[14,15]
  - Nonspecific neurologic/autonomic signs and constitutional symptoms. Tiredness, difficulty in concentration, and stiff neck.
- Aura (in MA)
  - Focal neurologic signs or symptoms: Visual (flashing lights), sensory (pins and needles), and motor (speech) symptoms.
  - Develop over 5 to 20 minutes and last for less than 60 minutes.
  - Followed in about 10 minutes by a typical headache.[16]
- Headache phase
  - See summary later in this article.
- Postdrome
  - Depressed, irritable, and tired.

Migraine Without Aura

Most common form of migraine.[1]

Summary of features of the headache phase

- Typically unilateral; no side preference.
  - Side-locked migraine in up to half of migraineurs.[17]
  - Bilateral in some patients.[17–19]
- Usually ocular, temporal, and frontal regions.[17]
  - Also occipital and neck regions.[17]
- Throbbing or pulsating; occasionally pressing.[19–21]
- Moderate to severe intensity.[9]
  - Not uniform.[21]
- Sharp periorbital "ice-pick" pains[22] interictally.
- Routine physical activity aggravates pain.[19,20]
  - Moving the head or coughing will accentuate headaches.
- Headache is insidious, may take 0.5 to 2.0 hours.[23]
- Periodic, typically lasting 4 to 72 hours.[1]
- Frequency is, in most cases, less than 1 per month[9,24,25] but may vary from up to 2 to 12 headaches per month.
- Vast majority report nausea and photophobia or phonophobia.[18,19]
  - 50% vomit during an attack.
- Autonomic signs (AS)
  - Usually lacrimation ($\approx$50%), linked to severity.[26,27]

Migraine Triggers

Several factors have been reported as initiators of individual attacks in migraineurs, termed triggers or precipitating factors,[28] and are reported by up to 90% of migraineurs[29,30]:

- Anxiety and stress.[30,31]
- Fatigue, sleeping difficulties.
  - Occasionally woken from sleep by a migraine,[32] early morning.[33]
  - Interestingly, sleeping may abolish headache.[32]
- Foods and drinks.
- Menstruation.
  - Hormone variations[34] associated with migraine onset and patterns.
  - A quarter of women report menstrually related migraine,[35,36] more so in clinic-based populations.[29,37,38]
  - Improvement or resolution of migraine headaches during late pregnancy.[20,39]
- Weather changes.
- Smells, smoke, and light.[40]

Differential Diagnosis

- Tension-type headache (TTH)
  - Clinical overlap with mild MWA is prominent.[41]
- Oral/Dental
  - Neurovascular pain in the lower face/oral cavity reported.[42,43]
    - Termed facial migraine, lower-half facial migraine or neurovascular orofacial pain.[42–45]
- Sinusitis
  - Extremely common misdiagnosis, particularly in migraines with midface pain.[46,47]
- Vascular disorders
  - Transient ischemic attacks, thromboembolic stroke, intracranial hematoma, subarachnoid hemorrhage, and arterial hypertension may cause migrainelike headaches.[48]
- Intracranial tumors, infections and regional trauma may induce migrainelike headaches.
- Some are sudden-onset headaches or are accompanied by atypical neurologic signs and symptoms.
  - See indications for neuroimaging in headaches.[49,50]
- Cervicogenic headache may clinically resemble migraine.

Chronic Migraine

Some migraine sufferers may have a clinically progressive disease in which migraine episodes increase in frequency over time.[51,52] A proportion of migraineurs (15.6%) describe daily or near-daily headaches[21] and approximately 2.5% of the general population has chronic migraine (CM). MWA is most prone to accelerate with frequent use of symptomatic medication, resulting in medication-overuse headache.[1] However, limited data are at our disposal to predict which patients will progress from episodic to CM.[52] The risk increases significantly in whites, with obesity and a high baseline headache frequency.[53,54]

Summary of CM features

- Bilateral; frontotemporal region.
  - Up to half may be strictly unilateral.[55,56]

- Mostly mild to moderate.
- Dull, pressing quality.[55]
- Occurs more than15 days per month (>3 months) with no medication overuse.[1]
  - Truly continuous headache in fewer than half of patients.
    - Superimposed, severe typical migraine attacks occur.[55,56]
- Nighttime arousals due to headache reported, particularly by women.[55,56]
- Most cases seem to begin as episodic migraine and transform.[57,58]
  - Many patients report episodic migraine that at approximately age 30 to 40 became increasingly frequent.
- Particularly in women, CM is still accompanied by mild migrainous features.[55,59]
- Menstrual relation and other triggers may still be prominent.[55,59]

Anxiety and depression seem to be common in patients with CM, affecting from one-third to nearly 90% of patients.[55] Hypothalamic dysfunction has been found in CM.[60]

Migraine Comorbidity

Strong evidence suggests a relation between migraine and depression or anxiety, stroke (particularly in MA with smoking), other pain syndromes, and allergies.[61,62]

Pathophysiology

Migraine is considered to be a result of a primary brain dysfunction, particularly in brainstem structures, that leads to activation and sensitization of the trigeminovascular system. The detailed pathophysiology of migraine is beyond the scope of this article. The reader is referred to pertinent reviews.[63,64]

Migraine Treatment

Although there is no cure, adequate control can be achieved for most migraineurs.

Nonpharmacologic treatment
- Patient education
  - Accurate, comprehensible information on importance of contributing factors, such as sleep, diet, and other lifestyle practices that may precipitate attacks.[65]

Pharmacologic treatment
- Abortive (acute, symptomatic).
  - Aim to rapidly relieve headache with no recurrence or side effects.
  - Used when fewer than 4 to 8 attacks per month or to supplement prophylactic regimens.
  - Nonspecific medication (**Table 1**).
    - Complementary treatments, such as butterbur, feverfew, and coenzyme-Q, may also be effective.[66]
  - Triptans (see **Table 1**)
    - Triptans of choice.[67]
      - Rizatriptan 10 mg consistently provides rapid relief.[67,68]
      - Almotriptan (12.5 mg) has good efficacy and tolerability.
      - Eletriptan will provide high efficacy with low recurrence but low tolerability.[68]
      - Frovatriptan for the prevention of menstrually related migraine.[69–71]

Table 1
Some of the common abortive treatments for migraine

Class	Drugs	Initial Oral Dose, mg
Analgesics	Aspirin	500–1000
Combinations	Aspirin and	500–600
	Paracetamol and	200–400
	Caffeine	50–200
	Paracetamol and	400
	Codeine	25
Ergot alkaloids	Dihydroergotamine NS	2
NSAIDs:		
Nonspecific	Naproxen sodium	550–825
	Ibuprofen	400–800
	Diclofenac	50–100
Selective COX 2 inhibitors	Rofecoxib	25–50
Triptans (5HT agonist)	Sumatriptan	50–100
	Sumatriptan NS	20 (1 NS metered dose)
	Sumatriptan SC	6
	Naratriptan	2.5
	Eletriptan	40
	Rizatriptan	10
	Zolmitriptan	2.5
	Zolmitriptan NS	2.5 (1 NS metered dose)
	Frovatriptan[a]	2.5
Opioids	Butorphanol NS	1–2 metered doses

Abbreviations: NS, nasal spray; NSAIDs, nonsteroidal anti inflammatory drugs; SC, subcutaneous injection.
[a] Schedule to prevent menstrually related migraines: 2.5 mg for 6 days during the perimenstrual period, loading dose of 2–4 tablets on day 1, followed by twice-daily frovatriptan 2.5 mg.

- Preventive (chronic, prophylactic; **Table 2**).
  - Aims to reduce attack frequency, severity, and duration.[72]
  - Use in frequent (>4–8 attacks monthly) or debilitating attacks.[72,73]
    - Early and aggressive treatment of frequent migraine is indicated.[74,75]
  - Drugs with high efficacy and mild to moderate adverse events.
    - β-blockers.
    - Amitriptyline.
    - Divalproex (good in CM).
    - Topiramate.[70,72,76]
    - Choice influenced by medical contraindications or comorbidities, such as insomnia, depression, and hypertension.[77]
  - Drugs with lower efficacy and mild to moderate adverse events.
    - Selective serotonin reuptake inhibitors, calcium channel antagonists, gabapentin, riboflavin, and nonsteroidal anti-inflammatory drugs (NSAIDs).[77]

Treatment Outcome
- About two-thirds of patients will experience a 50% reduction in headache frequency on most preventive therapies.[78]
  - Better rate for sodium valproate.[79]

In summary, migraine is a debilitating syndrome that in mild or atypical forms is often misdiagnosed. Correct diagnosis allows the control of most headaches.

Table 2
Choice of migraine preventive treatment

Drug	Dose, mg	Adverse Events	Contraindications	Relative Indications
Propranolol (SR)	80–240	Bradycardia Hypotension Fatigue Sleep disturbances Dyspepsia Depression	Asthma Depression Cardiac failure Raynaud disease Diabetes	Hypertension Angina
Amitriptyline	10–50	Sedation Weight gain Dry mouth Blurred vision Constipation Urinary retention Postural hypotension	Mania Urinary retention Heart block	Insomnia Anxiety Depression TTH Other chronic pains
Sodium valproate	500–1000	Nausea, vomiting Alopecia Tremor Weight gain/loss	Liver disease Bleeding disorder	Mania Epilepsy Anxiety
Topiramate	25–200	Dizziness, confusion, language problems, paresthesias, nausea, anorexia, diplopia	Renal disease, Respiratory disorders Glaucoma	Overweight

The 4 most effective or commonly used drugs are presented. Choice is influenced by adverse events, comorbidity, and relative indications. The efficacy of all 4 drugs is similar.
Abbreviation: TTH, tension-type headache.

TACS

TACs are primary headaches with a common clinical phenotype consisting of trigeminal pain and AS.

Pathophysiology of TACS

The current pathophysiologic model attempts to explain the 3 major features of the TACs: trigeminal pain, rhythmicity (particularly in CH), and autonomic signs. Taken together, current data suggest that CH and other TACs are conditions whose pathophysiological basis is in the central nervous system, including the hypothalamus, which drives the initiation of the clinical phenotype. Detailed description of the pathophysiology is beyond the scope of this article; see Refs.[80–82]

CH

CH is the archetypal TAC, with severe pain and major autonomic activation.[1] The precise genetics of CH are unclear. However, first-degree relatives of patients with CH are up to 14 to 48 times and second-degree relatives are 2 to 8 times more likely to have CH than the general population.[82] CH is likely to have an autosomal dominant gene with low penetrance.[82]

CH typically appears between the ages of 20 and 29 years[83] and is more common than previously thought: 53 cases per 100,000[84] but may reach 120 to 300 per 100,000[85] and seems to affect men more than women.

A unique feature of episodic CH is the distinctive circadian and circannual periodicity. Episodic CH commonly occurs at least once daily for a period of weeks, at the same time of day or night.[83] Active periods (6–12 weeks) are followed by a temporary remission that may last from weeks to years (average 12 months). Attacks tend to be shorter and less severe at the beginning and toward the end of each cluster period. At its initial onset, CH active periods are seasonal, occurring around spring or autumn.[86]

There are 2 distinct temporal presentations of CH; most (80%–85%) suffer from the episodic type, characterized by at least 2 cluster periods separated by pain-free periods of 1 month or more over 7 to 365 days.[1] In chronic CH, repeated attacks recur over more than a year without remission or with remission periods lasting less than 1 month. Interictal pain may also be present between attacks or between clusters.[87] Of the 15% of patients with chronic CH, in two-thirds it usually begins as such and in the remaining evolves from the episodic form. Up to half of patients with chronic CH report transition to an episodic pattern.[88] Over the course of the disease, attack duration tends to lengthen in both episodic and chronic CH.

Surprisingly for such a dramatic syndrome, the interval until final diagnosis was 3 to 6 years: 34% to 45% had consulted a dentist and 27% to 33% had consulted an otolaryngologist before accurate diagnosis.[87,89–92] Among factors that increased the diagnostic delay were referral patterns, the presence of migrainous features, an episodic attack pattern, and a young age at onset.

Summary of CH features
The IHS requires at least 5 attacks that meet the criteria outlined.

- Periorbital or ocular[86] pain.
  - "Lower" and "upper" subtypes of CH:
    - Upper CH: forehead, temporal, and parietal regions.[93]
    - Lower CH: temporal, and suboccipital with radiation to the teeth, jaws, neck,[93] teeth, and cheeks.[87,94]
- Unilateral.
  - 20% of cases may change sides.[86]
  - Attacks alternate sides; more common between clusters than between attacks in the same cluster.[86]
- Excruciating severity.
  - Rated as 8 to 10 on a 10-point visual analog scale (VAS) by more than 85% of patients and some report considering suicide.[86]
- Pain is nonspecific: throbbing or boring, burning, stabbing.[95]
  - "Hot poker" or a "stabbing" feeling in the eye.[94]
  - Sudden jabs of intense pain often felt.
- Accompanied by at least 1 of the following ipsilateral autonomic signs:
  - Conjunctival injection/lacrimation
  - Nasal congestion/rhinorrhea
  - Eyelid edema
  - Forehead/facial sweating
  - Miosis and ptosis
  - Restlessness (not a local autonomic sign but frequent [>80%]).
    - Patients appear agitated, continually move around, particularly during severe attacks[96]; in sharp contrast to the quiet-seeking behavior observed in migraine.
- Lasts 15 to 180 minutes
  - Peak intensity is usually rapid: within 3 minutes but may take 9 to 10 minutes.[95]
  - Long-lasting attacks are rare, but may last from 3 to 48 hours.[87]
- Frequency of 1 every other day to 8 per day.

Additional features

- Nocturnal CH is high particularly prevalent (51%–73%).
  - Pain awakens patients within 90 minutes; the onset of rapid eye movement (REM) sleep.[94]
    - Association between episodic chronic CH and REM sleep less established.[97]
  - Patients with CH significantly suffer from obstructive sleep apnea.[98]
- Alcohol may precipitate CH attacks during active cluster periods.[99]
  - Some patients with chronic CH report high alcohol/tobacco consumption.[100]
- CH prodromes include AS and mild pain or nonpainful sensations in the area that subsequently becomes painful.[101]
  - Blurred vision, sensitivity to smells, nausea, dyspepsia, hunger, irritability, tiredness, and tenseness.[101]
  - Premonitory symptoms may predict CH days before onset, present in 40% of CH cases.
    - Similar to those experienced by migraineurs.[101]
      - "Auralike" symptoms in 14% of cases.[102]

Autonomic signs

- Ipsilateral lacrimation most frequent AS; in approximately 90% of cases.[94]
  - Common and pronounced in CH, subtler in other TACs.
  - Rarely ptosis and miosis (partial Horner syndrome) may persist.
  - Intensity of AS may be related to pain severity.[103]
- Migrainous features are common in CH.[104]
  - Photophobia, phonophobia, nausea, and vomiting in up to half of cases.
    - Phonophobia and photophobia are unilateral: in migraine bilateral.[105]
- CH associated with transient hemiparesis, visual symptoms, photophobia, phonophobia, and nausea.[104]
  - Strikingly similar to side-locked migraine.

Differential diagnosis and secondary CH

- Dental/Sinus pathology
  - May be related to referral patterns[87,89–92] and occurrence of "lower CH."[93]

Occur as a result of rare pathologies:
- Vascular lesions, multiple sclerosis,[86] pituitary tumor,[106] trauma.[107]
- Secondary TACs have no "typical" presentation; mimic primary TAC.[108,109]
  - Neuroimaging must be performed for all TACs or atypical[108,110,111] TAC-like syndromes.[112]

CH treatment

Nonpharmacologic treatment
- A clear explanation of mechanisms, treatment options, and prognosis (**Tables 3–5**).
- Based on attack patterns, patients avoid daytime naps.
- Avoid alcoholic beverages and other triggers.
- Altitude hypoxemia may trigger an attack during active periods, but may be pharmacologically prevented.[113]

Table 3
Selected abortive pharmacologic treatment options for episodic cluster headache

Agent	Dose	Comments	Side Effects
Oxygen (inhaled via face mask)	5–10 L/min 15 min 15 L/min may be tried	First line but cumbersome. Hyperbaric oxygen also efficacious but impractical.	None
Sumatriptan	6–12 mg SC	First line, fast, and efficacious; 12 mg as effective as 6 mg but with more side effects. Marginally less effective in chronic CH.	Contraindicated in CV disease. Fatigue Nausea/vomiting Chest symptoms Skin reactions over puncture wound.
	20 mg IN	Less effective but easier to use.	Contraindicated in CV disease. IN<SC
Zolmitriptan	5–10 mg IN	Limited efficacy, alternative to IN sumatriptan.	Contraindicated in CV disease. Better in episodic CH.
Dihydroergotamine	0.5–1.0 mg IN (bilateral)	Reduces severity but not frequency. Risk of rebound.	Contraindicated in CV disease. Do not use with a triptan.
Lignocaine	1 mL of 4%–10% solution applied IN on cotton pledget bilaterally	Pain is decreased but not enough studies. Needs to be inserted deep near pterygopalatine foramen.	Bitter taste

Abbreviations: CH, cluster headache; CV, cardiovascular; IN, intranasal; SC, subcutaneous injection.

Nonpharmacologic treatment[114,115]

- Abortive (first line)[114]
  - Rapid symptomatic relief with oxygen inhalation.[114]
    - Useful diagnostic test.
    - In resistant cases try higher flow rates (15 L/min).[116]
  - Subcutaneous sumatriptan if medically fit.
- Transitional and prophylactic[114]
  - Rapid transitional prophylaxis may be attained with corticosteroids.
    - For a limited period in selected patients.[117]
  - Long-term prophylaxis usually with verapamil[113] in both episodic and chronic CH.
    - Topiramate as second-line therapy.
    - Although many side effects, lithium carbonate may be considered.
- Surgical,[118] for carefully selected recalcitrant cases.

Recent reports indicate that medication overuse headache (MOH) is a possible complication in patients with CH and patients with other TACs.[119,120] Remission periods in many patients may increase with time, and beyond the age of 65 to 75, active CH is rare.

Table 4
Prophylactic treatment of episodic cluster headache

Agent	Target Dose	Comments	Side Effects
Verapamil	160–480 mg/d (PO)	First-line treatment. Perform baseline and 6 monthly ECGs.	Hypotension, bradycardia, heart block, dizziness, and fatigue
Prednisone	80 mg (PO) Typical schedule: 80 mg first 2 d. Reduce by 20 mg every 2 d. Reduce to 10 mg/d for last 2 d	Good for initial and transitional therapy until, eg, verapamil takes effect. Prolonged use not recommended because of side effects. Taper over 10–21 d.	Increased appetite, nervousness, hyperglycemia, insomnia, headaches
Topiramate	25–200 mg/d (PO)	Increase by 25 mg/d every 5 d.	Cognitive effects, paresthesias, dizziness
Valproic acid	600–2000 mg/d (PO)	Efficacious in patients with pronounced migrainous features. Monitor liver function.	Nausea, dizziness, dyspepsia, thrombocytopenia
Gabapentin	900 mg/d (PO)	Few studies but promising results.	Drowsiness
Melatonin	9–10 mg/d nocte (PO)	Few studies.	None

Abbreviations: ECG, electrocardiogram; nocte, nighttime; PO, orally.

PH

PH is rare, with an estimated prevalence of 2 to 20 per 100,000.[85,121–123] Mean age of onset is usually 34 to 41 years, but children aged 6 and adults aged 81 years have been reported with average illness duration of 13 years.[124–126] The episodic form is considered to have an earlier mean age of onset (27 years) than the chronic form (37 years).[124]

Only 20% of PHs behave episodically,[125] and many of these eventually develop into a chronic form.[124] The IHS requires at least 20 attacks that meet the criteria outlined.

Table 5
Treatment of chronic cluster headache

Agent	Target Dose	Comments	Side Effects
Verapamil	360–480 mg/d (PO)	First-line treatment. Perform baseline ECG.	Hypotension, bradycardia, heart block, dizziness, and fatigue
Lithium carbonate	300–900 mg (PO)	Requires monitoring of renal and thyroid function, and of serum concentrations (best at 0.4–0.8 mEq/L).	Weakness, nausea, tremor, slurred speech, blurred vision *Side effects > verapamil.*

Abbreviations: ECG, electrocardiogram; PO, orally.

Summary of PH features

- Unilateral, severe orbital, or periorbital pain.
  - Rarely may become bilateral.[127]
  - Also temporal, periauricular, maxillary, and, rarely, occipital areas.[125,128]
  - Referral to the shoulder, neck, and arm is quite common.[128]
  - Strong pain may cross the midline.
  - The vast majority of attacks do not change sides.[125]
- Last 2 to 30 minutes.
  - More usually 13 to 29 minutes, but may last nearly an hour.
  - Pain onset is rapid and mostly peaks in less than 5 minutes.[125]
- Sharp and excruciating.[125]
  - Also throbbing, stabbing, sharp, or boring.[125,129]
- Accompanied by at least 1 of the following ipsilateral autonomic signs:
  - Conjunctival injection/lacrimation
  - Nasal congestion/rhinorrhea
  - Eyelid edema
  - Forehead/facial sweating
  - Miosis and ptosis
- More than 5 attacks daily.
  - Usually 8 to 30 attacks per 24 hours.[124]
  - Seasonal pattern of attacks in PH patients has been described.[130]
  - The temporal similarity to CH behavior has led to the term "modified cluster pattern."[128]
  - 30% report REM-related[131] nocturnal attacks that wake.[124]
- Absolute response to indomethacin.

Additional features

AS may occur bilaterally but are more pronounced on the symptomatic side. The most commonly seen are ipsilateral lacrimation, nasal congestion, conjunctival injection, and rhinnorrhea.[129,132] In patient series, one "migrainous feature" was reported by nearly 90% of cases.[125,133]

Secondary paroxysmal hemicrania

- Malignancy, central nervous system disease, and benign tumors.[110]
- Parotid gland epidermoid carcinoma with cerebral metastasis.[134]
- Systemic diseases.[110,124]
- All PH cases require imaging.[135]

Treatment

The response of PH to indomethacin is absolute. Most cases respond within 24 hours, but 3 days at 75 mg followed, if needed, by 150 mg for a further 3 days is recommended as trial therapy[136]; high persistent dosage requirements may indicate underlying pathology. Prognosis in PH is good and long-term remission has been reported.[137] Indomethacin-resistant PH may respond to topiramate.[112,138,139] A summary of therapies for PH, SUNCT, and HC is shown in **Table 6**.

SUNCT

SUNCT syndrome is a unilateral headache/facial pain characterized by brief paroxysmal attacks accompanied by ipsilateral local AS, usually conjunctival injection and lacrimation.[140] The similarities of this syndrome to trigeminal neuralgia (TN) are

Table 6
Pharmacotherapy of PH, SUNCT, and HC

Headache	Drug of Choice	Target Dose (Route)	Second Line
PH	Indomethacin	75–225 mg/d (PO)	Other NSAIDs Verapamil Acetazolamide
SUNCT	Lamotrigine	100–300 mg/d (PO)	Gabapentin 900–2700 mg/d Topiramate 50–200 mg/d
HC	Indomethacin	25–300 mg/d (PO)	Other NSAIDs Piroxicam-beta-cyclodextrin

Abbreviations: HC, hemicrania continua; NSAID, nonsteroidal anti-inflammatory drug; PH, parox-ysmal hemicranias; PO, orally; SUNCT, short-lasting neuralgiform headache attacks with conjunc-tival injection and tearing.

marked, particularly the triggering mechanism and many believe SUNCT to be a TN variant.[141]

Estimates suggest SUNCT/short-lasting, unilateral, neuralgiform headache attacks with cranial autonomic features (SUNA) to be as common as PH.[85] SUNCT is presently considered only slightly more common in men,[142,143] with a mean onset at approxi-mately 50 years.[142,144] SUNCT occurring in siblings has recently been presented as "familial SUNCT."[145] The IHS requires at least 20 attacks that meet the criteria outlined.

Clinical features of SUNCT

- Unilateral, ocular/periocular pain,[1] but may involve most head areas.[146]
  - Pain spreading across the midline or changing sides is rare.[142]
- Moderate to severe pain[142]; less severe than TN.
- Pain accompanied by ipsilateral conjunctival injection and lacrimation.
- Usually stabbing or pulsating.
  - Sometimes electric or burning.[142]
- Lasts from 5 to 240 seconds.
  - Usually 15 to 120 seconds (mean 1 minute).
  - Longer attacks of up to 10 minutes and even 2 to 3 hours reported.[147]
  - "SUNCT status"; (rare) pain most of the day for 1 to 3 days.[148]
  - Low-grade background pain/discomfort occurs.[148]
- Three patterns of attacks described.[112,146]
  - Classical single attacks.
  - Groups of a number of stabs/attacks.
  - "Saw-tooth" pattern with numerous stabs/attacks lasting minutes.
- Frequency is from 3 to 200 daily.
  - Inconsistent and irregular; average of 28 per day.[147]
  - A bimodal distribution of attacks occurring in the morning and late afternoon has been observed.
  - Fewer than 2% of attacks occur at night.[147]
  - A "clusterlike" pattern has been reported with active and inactive periods.[140]
  - A seasonal pattern has been reported in SUNA.[149]

Additional features

Pain in SUNCT may be triggered by light mechanical stimuli in the areas innervated by the trigeminal nerve but with a short latency until pain onset.[142] Extratrigeminal triggers, including neck movements, have also been shown to precipitate attacks. No refractory period has been demonstrated in SUNCT.[142,150]

By definition, SUNCT is accompanied by marked ipsilateral conjunctival injection and lacrimation that appear rapidly with onset of pain.[1] Nasal stuffiness and rhinorrhea are common; sweating may accompany attacks but is rare and often subclinical.[140,151]

SUNA

This is a relatively novel diagnostic entity included in the IHS classification's appendix. Essentially 2 criteria differentiate it from SUNCT: SUNA may be accompanied by any autonomic sign (eg, nasal congestion), and attack duration has been extended to up until 10 minutes.[1,112,120,146]

Secondary SUNCT/SUNA

- Brainstem infarction.
- Cerebellopontine region: arteriovenous malformations, astrocytoma, or other tumors/cysts.
- Cavernous hemangioma of the brainstem.
- Cavernous sinus tumor, extraorbital cystic mass, vertebral artery dissection, and neurofibromatosis.[110,142,152,153]
- Posttraumatic.[142]
- All patients with SUNCT should be referred for imaging.[142]

SUNCT/SUNA treatment

- Lamotrigine is the drug of choice (see **Table 6**).[112,154]
  - Initial dosage is 25 mg per day; increase very slowly, reach target in 7 or more weeks.
- SUNCT may respond to steroids.[155]
- Anticonvulsant drugs may produce some improvement.
  - Carbamazepine, topiramate, and gabapentin (see **Table 6**).[112]
- Case reports of successful surgical microvascular decompression and percutaneous trigeminal ganglion compression for SUNCT.[156]
- Remissions have been observed and may last for several months.[157,158]

HC

As HC is further reported, this headache entity is increasingly considered a TAC variant.[1] As in other TACs, HC seems to be often misdiagnosed and mistreated; in a recent series, time to correct diagnosis was 5 years.[159]

Clinical features of HC

- Unilateral headache for more than 3 months.
  - Pain in the frontal and temporal regions and periorbitally.[160]
  - Although *very rare*, pain can also change sides.[161] Few bilateral cases.
- Daily and continuous pain.
- Severity is moderate (VAS 4.7).[162]
  - Characterized (74%) by fluctuations in pain severity.
  - Exacerbations are totally disabling in about 40% of patients.[162]
  - Exacerbations result in severe pain (VAS 9.3) lasting 30 minutes to 10 hours and even up to 2 to 5 days.[86,162]
  - During exacerbation, HC is almost indistinguishable from migraine.[162]
  - Patients may report a sharp pain similar to the condition of "jabs and jolts."[162]

- ○ Some patients (18%) describe a distinct ocular sensation mimicking a foreign body (or sand), that may accompany or precede the headaches.[86]
- Pain is throbbing (one-third of cases); may appear as pain intensity increases.[86,162]
- Complete response to indomethacin.
- During exacerbations, accompanied by at least 1 of the following ipsilateral autonomic phenomena/signs:
  - ○ Conjunctival injection/lacrimation
  - ○ Nasal congestion/rhinorrhea
  - ○ Miosis and ptosis

Additional features

Two forms of HC have been described: remitting and continuous. The remitting form is characterized by headache that can last for some days followed by a pain-free period lasting from 2 to 15 days.[86,162] One-third of remitting cases become continuous following a mean duration of 7.8 years.[86,162] Nocturnal attacks were reported in up to half of patients.[86,162]

HC is not usually accompanied by notable pathology or other abnormalities.[86] Most published cases of HC with computerized scanning of the head, neurologic and other physical examination, hematology, and serum biochemistry were all normal. Cases of HC secondary to pathology or systemic disease have been reported.[110]

There is usually a paucity of AS in HC. However, during exacerbation, AS commonly appear singly or in various combinations, but are still relatively mild. This strengthens the hypothesis that activation of AS is dependent on pain severity. The most common signs present in 30% to 40% of patients are photophobia, nausea, conjunctival injection, phonophobia, and tearing.[86] During exacerbations up to 60% of patients display qualities such as photophobia, phonophobia, nausea, and, more rarely, vomiting.[162] HC with aura has also been described, further linking HC to migraine pathophysiology.[163] More rarely (15%–18%) nasal stuffiness or rhinorrhea, vomiting, or ptosis may also be reported.[86] These features establish the HC phenotype as straddling both TACs and migraine.

Secondary hemicrania continua

- Medication abuse.[86]
- Mesenchymal tumor in the sphenoid bone has been reported.[86]
- Head trauma and surgery.[86,162]

Treatment

- Indomethacin totally effective.[1]
  - ○ Relief occurs within hours or 1 to 2 days.
- Other NSAIDs are less effective.[164]
- Piroxicam-beta-cyclodextrin is a good alternative for selected cases.[165]

Differential diagnosis of TACs

Given the predominate sensory system involved, referral patterns of TACs often involve orofacial structures and at times may primarily present in intraoral or unusual facial sites. Thus, CH and PH have caused misdiagnosis as dental pain leading to unnecessary dental interventions.[87,90,92,94] Cluster headaches are often seen by ear, nose, and throat surgeons and erroneously diagnosed as sinus pathology.[87,90,92,94]

TTHS

The IHS subclassifies TTH into episodic (infrequent and frequent), chronic, and probable TTH. The individual attacks in these subentities have similar clinical features with some subtle differences; severity and the occurrence of mild nausea tend to increase with frequency. Pericranial muscle tenderness is an extremely common feature in patients with TTH, but because some patients do not demonstrate this feature, the IHS subclassifies TTH as with or without pericranial tenderness.

TTH is extremely common, and most individuals will have experienced one in their lifetime.[166] TTH has a 1-year prevalence in adults of more than 80%, higher than migraine.[166,167] Infrequent episodic TTH (IETTH), which occurs on average once per month, is most common (48%–59%) but does not usually require medical attention.[168,169] One-year prevalence of frequent episodic TTH (FETTH) is 18% to 43% and 10% to 25% report weekly headaches.[169,170] TTH, in particular chronic TTH (CTTH), is thought to account for more than 10% of disease-related absenteeism.[171]

The average onset age of TTH is 20 to 30 years with peak prevalence in the third to fifth decades.[168] However, up to 25% of school children report having TTH,[172] and in the older population (>60 years) the prevalence is 20% to 30%.

Genetic studies reveal that first-degree relatives of CTTH sufferers are 3 times as likely to also suffer headaches relative to the population.[173] FETTH is significantly affected by environmental factors, with evidence for only a minor genetic contribution.[174]

Episodic Tension-Type Headache

Clinical features

- Bilateral in >90%.
- Occipital, parietal, temporal or frontal areas.[19,175]
  - "Bandlike" or "caplike."
  - Site may vary with intensity.[175]
- Pressurelike, dull or tight.[175]
  - Throbbing is rare and related to severity.[175,176]
- Intensity is mild to moderate.[19,177]
  - Increases with headache frequency.[178]
- Duration 30 minutes to 7 days.[179]
- 25% of episodic TTH (ETTH) evolves into CTTH.[170,180]
- Sleep disturbances.[181]
- Mild to moderate anorexia.[19]
- Occasional and mild photophobia (10%) or phonophobia (7%).[19,175]

Many patients will suffer both migraines and TTH, which may further affect quality of life. Interestingly, ETTH in migraine sufferers responds to sumatriptan, a migraine-specific drug, whereas in patients who do not suffer from migraine, it does not.[182] This may suggest that mild migraines may phenotypically be very similar to ETTH.

ETTH is commonly precipitated by a number of factors: stress, fatigue, disturbed meals, menstruation, alcohol, and a lack of sleep.[31,40] Although TTH is usually not aggravated by physical activity,[175] there are reports that in some patients with TTH, exercise may aggravate pain.[183,184]

Other than in location, TTH is very similar to masticatory myofascial pain.

CTTH

CTTH is one of the subtypes of a group simply termed "chronic daily headaches," based on the daily or near daily occurrence of headaches.

Clinical features of CTTH

Classically, the patient with CTTH is middle-aged and female, with a long headache history that began with episodic headaches 10 to 20 years previously and slowly increased in frequency.[54,58,185] The clinical features of CTTH are largely similar to those in FETTH, with differences in accompanying features, treatment response, and impact on quality of life.

- CTTH is bilateral.
  - Frontal, temporal, or frontotemporal regions.[19,58,186]
- Pressurelike.[19]
- Mostly moderate pain.
  - <10% severe.[19,187]
- Continuous or daily headache.
  - Mean frequency is 23 to 30 headache days per month.[186,188]
- Increased pericranial tenderness.[189]
- Photophobia or phonophobia.[190]
- Physical activity may worsen pain in some patients with CTTH.[19,187]
- Depression, anxiety, and lack of sleep common.[191]

Pathophysiology

Interrelationships between peripheral and central mechanisms probably underlie the initiation of TTHs, but the exact etiology is uncertain.[192,193] The evidence suggests that peripheral mechanisms play a major role in ETTHs, whereas central mechanisms, such as faulty inhibitory mechanisms and central sensitization, are prominent in CTTH.[194] It is interesting to note that the same etiologic factors are considered in TTH and in masticatory myofascial pain (MMP), further suggesting common pathophysiology.

Treatment of TTH

- Pharmacologic
  - Abortive therapy
    - 800 mg ibuprofen or 825 mg naproxen.[195]
    - 1 g of paracetamol.[196]
    - Triptans for CTTH, or mixed migraine and ETTH.[197,198]
  - Prophylactic
    - Tricyclic antidepressants are efficacious.[199]
      - Effective in CTTH but not in ETTH.
      - 10 mg daily taken just before bedtime and then titrated.
        - CTTH may need up to 75 mg.[200]
    - Muscle relaxants and botulinum toxin,[201] mixed results.

Nonpharmacological interventions

- Behavioral.[202]
  - Relaxation training.
    - Relaxation and electromyographic biofeedback therapies are effective mainly in ETTH.[203]
  - Biofeedback training.
  - Cognitive-behavioral (stress-management) therapy.
    - In patients with CTTH, the combination of stress management with a tricyclic antidepressant (amitriptyline $\leq$100 mg/d, or nortriptyline $\leq$75 mg/d) induced significant reductions in headache index scores than each therapy alone or placebo.[204]

- o Physiotherapy, massage therapy, acupuncture, or chiropractic manipulation may be beneficial for TTH, but the evidence is weak.[205]
- Temporomandibular disorder therapies.
  - o Occlusal splints or physiotherapy.[206]
    - Reduction in severity and frequency of headaches.
  - o No significant effect of occlusal adjustment was observed on headache frequency.[207]

REFERENCES

1. The International classification of headache disorders. 2nd edition. 2004. Available at: http://ihs-classification.org/en/. Accessed October 9, 2011.
2. Henry P, Michel P, Brochet B, et al. A nationwide survey of migraine in France: prevalence and clinical features in adults. GRIM. Cephalalgia 1992;12(4): 229–37 [discussion: 186].
3. O'Brien B, Goeree R, Streiner D. Prevalence of migraine headache in Canada: a population-based survey. Int J Epidemiol 1994;23(5):1020–6.
4. Stewart WF, Lipton RB, Celentano DD, et al. Prevalence of migraine headache in the United States. Relation to age, income, race, and other sociodemographic factors. JAMA 1992;267(1):64–9.
5. Rasmussen BK, Jensen R, Schroll M, et al. Epidemiology of headache in a general population—a prevalence study. J Clin Epidemiol 1991;44(11):1147–57.
6. Olesen J. The migraines: introduction. In: Olesen J, Tfelt-Hansen P, Welch KM, editors. The headaches. 2nd edition. Philadelphia: Lippincott Williams & Wilkins; 2000. p. 223–5.
7. Cavallini A, Micieli G, Bussone G, et al. Headache and quality of life. Headache 1995;35(1):29–35.
8. Steiner TJ. Headache burdens and bearers. Funct Neurol 2000;15(Suppl 3): 219–23.
9. Steiner TJ, Scher AI, Stewart WF, et al. The prevalence and disability burden of adult migraine in England and their relationships to age, gender and ethnicity. Cephalalgia 2003;23(7):519–27.
10. Russell MB, Olesen J. Increased familial risk and evidence of genetic factor in migraine. BMJ 1995;311(7004):541–4.
11. Stewart WF, Staffa J, Lipton RB, et al. Familial risk of migraine: a population-based study. Ann Neurol 1997;41(2):166–72.
12. Estevez M, Gardner KL. Update on the genetics of migraine. Hum Genet 2004; 114(3):225–35.
13. Mochi M, Cevoli S, Cortelli P, et al. A genetic association study of migraine with dopamine receptor 4, dopamine transporter and dopamine-beta-hydroxylase genes. Neurol Sci 2003;23(6):301–5.
14. Giffin NJ, Ruggiero L, Lipton RB, et al. Premonitory symptoms in migraine: an electronic diary study. Neurology 2003;60(6):935–40.
15. Kelman L. The premonitory symptoms (prodrome): a tertiary care study of 893 migraineurs. Headache 2004;44(9):865–72.
16. Kelman L. The aura: a tertiary care study of 952 migraine patients. Cephalalgia 2004;24(9):728–34.
17. Kelman L. Migraine pain location: a tertiary care study of 1283 migraineurs. Headache 2005;45(8):1038–47.
18. Rasmussen BK, Olesen J. Migraine with aura and migraine without aura: an epidemiological study. Cephalalgia 1992;12(4):221–8 [discussion: 186].

19. Rasmussen BK, Jensen R, Olesen J. A population-based analysis of the diagnostic criteria of the International Headache Society. Cephalalgia 1991;11(3):129–34.
20. Russell MB, Rasmussen BK, Fenger K, et al. Migraine without aura and migraine with aura are distinct clinical entities: a study of four hundred and eighty-four male and female migraineurs from the general population. Cephalalgia 1996;16(4):239–45.
21. Stewart WF, Lipton RB, Kolodner K. Migraine disability assessment (MIDAS) score: relation to headache frequency, pain intensity, and headache symptoms. Headache 2003;43(3):258–65.
22. Rasmussen BK, Olesen J. Symptomatic and nonsymptomatic headaches in a general population. Neurology 1992;42(6):1225–31.
23. Zagami AS, Rasmussen BK. Symptomatology of migraine. In: Olesen J, Tfelt-Hansen P, Welch KM, editors. The headaches. 2nd edition. Philadelphia: Lippincott Williams and Wilkins; 2000. p. 337–43.
24. Pryse-Phillips W, Findlay H, Tugwell P, et al. A Canadian population survey on the clinical, epidemiologic and societal impact of migraine and tension-type headache. Can J Neurol Sci 1992;19(3):333–9.
25. Rasmussen P. Facial pain. IV. A prospective study of 1052 patients with a view of: precipitating factors, associated symptoms, objective psychiatric and neurological symptoms. Acta Neurochir (Wien) 1991;108(3–4):100–9.
26. Barbanti P, Fabbrini G, Pesare M, et al. Unilateral cranial autonomic symptoms in migraine. Cephalalgia 2002;22(4):256–9.
27. Kaup AO, Mathew NT, Levyman C, et al. 'Side locked' migraine and trigeminal autonomic cephalgias: evidence for clinical overlap. Cephalalgia 2003;23(1):43–9.
28. Martin VT, Behbehani MM. Toward a rational understanding of migraine trigger factors. Med Clin North Am 2001;85(4):911–41.
29. Chabriat H, Danchot J, Michel P, et al. Precipitating factors of headache. A prospective study in a national control-matched survey in migraineurs and nonmigraineurs. Headache 1999;39(5):335–8.
30. Rasmussen BK. Migraine and tension-type headache in a general population: precipitating factors, female hormones, sleep pattern and relation to lifestyle. Pain 1993;53(1):65–72.
31. Spierings EL, Ranke AH, Honkoop PC. Precipitating and aggravating factors of migraine versus tension-type headache. Headache 2001;41(6):554–8.
32. Kelman L, Rains JC. Headache and sleep: examination of sleep patterns and complaints in a large clinical sample of migraineurs. Headache 2005;45(7):904–10.
33. Dodick DW, Eross EJ, Parish JM, et al. Clinical, anatomical, and physiologic relationship between sleep and headache. Headache 2003;43(3):282–92.
34. Granella F, Sances G, Allais G, et al. Characteristics of menstrual and nonmenstrual attacks in women with menstrually related migraine referred to headache centres. Cephalalgia 2004;24(9):707–16.
35. Couturier EG, Bomhof MA, Neven AK, et al. Menstrual migraine in a representative Dutch population sample: prevalence, disability and treatment. Cephalalgia 2003;23(4):302–8.
36. Martin VT, Wernke S, Mandell K, et al. Defining the relationship between ovarian hormones and migraine headache. Headache 2005;45(9):1190–201.
37. Granella F, Sances G, Pucci E, et al. Migraine with aura and reproductive life events: a case control study. Cephalalgia 2000;20(8):701–7.

38. Robbins L. Precipitating factors in migraine: a retrospective review of 494 patients. Headache 1994;34(4):214–6.
39. Rasmussen BK. Epidemiology of headache. Cephalalgia 2001;21(7):774–7.
40. Karli N, Zarifoglu M, Calisir N, et al. Comparison of pre-headache phases and trigger factors of migraine and episodic tension-type headache: do they share similar clinical pathophysiology? Cephalalgia 2005;25(6):444–51.
41. Zebenholzer K, Wober C, Kienbacher C, et al. Migrainous disorder and headache of the tension-type not fulfilling the criteria: a follow-up study in children and adolescents. Cephalalgia 2000;20(7):611–6.
42. Benoliel R, Elishoov H, Sharav Y. Orofacial pain with vascular-type features. Oral Surg Oral Med Oral Pathol Oral Radiol Endod 1997;84(5):506–12.
43. Penarrocha M, Bandres A, Penarrocha M, et al. Lower-half facial migraine: a report of 11 cases. J Oral Maxillofac Surg 2004;62(12):1453–6.
44. Daudia AT, Jones NS. Facial migraine in a rhinological setting. Clin Otolaryngol Allied Sci 2002;27(6):521–5.
45. Lance JW, Goadsby PJ. Mechanism and management of headache. 7th edition. Philadelphia: Elsevier; 2005.
46. Eross E, Dodick D, Eross M. The Sinus, Allergy and Migraine Study (SAMS). Headache 2007;47(2):213–24.
47. Schreiber CP, Hutchinson S, Webster CJ, et al. Prevalence of migraine in patients with a history of self-reported or physician-diagnosed "sinus" headache. Arch Intern Med 2004;164(16):1769–72.
48. Campbell JK, Sakai F. The migraines: diagnosis and differential diagnosis. In: Olesen J, Tfelt-Hansen P, Welch KM, editors. The headaches. 2nd edition. Philadelphia: Lippincott Williams & Wilkins; 2000.
49. Evidence-based guidelines in the primary care setting: neuroimaging in patients with nonacute headache. American Academy of Neurology; 2000. Available at: http://www.aan.com/professionals/practice/pdfs/gl0088.pdf. Accessed May 17, 2013.
50. Sandrini G, Friberg L, Janig W, et al. Neurophysiological tests and neuroimaging procedures in non-acute headache: guidelines and recommendations. Eur J Neurol 2004;11(4):217–24.
51. Lipton RB, Pan J. Is migraine a progressive brain disease? JAMA 2004;291(4): 493–4.
52. Lipton RB, Bigal ME. Migraine: epidemiology, impact, and risk factors for progression. Headache 2005;45(Suppl 1):S3–13.
53. Katsarava Z, Schneeweiss S, Kurth T, et al. Incidence and predictors for chronicity of headache in patients with episodic migraine. Neurology 2004;62(5): 788–90.
54. Scher AI, Stewart WF, Ricci JA, et al. Factors associated with the onset and remission of chronic daily headache in a population-based study. Pain 2003; 106(1–2):81–9.
55. Krymchantowski AV, Moreira PF. Clinical presentation of transformed migraine: possible differences among male and female patients. Cephalalgia 2001; 21(5):558–66.
56. Spierings EL, Schroevers M, Honkoop PC, et al. Presentation of chronic daily headache: a clinical study. Headache 1998;38(3):191–6.
57. Mathew NT, Reuveni U, Perez F. Transformed or evolutive migraine. Headache 1987;27(2):102–6.
58. Solomon S, Lipton RB, Newman LC. Clinical features of chronic daily headache. Headache 1992;32(7):325–9.

59. Srikiatkhachorn A, Phanthumchinda K. Prevalence and clinical features of chronic daily headache in a headache clinic. Headache 1997;37(5):277–80.
60. Peres MF, Sanchez del Rio M, Seabra ML, et al. Hypothalamic involvement in chronic migraine. J Neurol Neurosurg Psychiatry 2001;71(6):747–51.
61. Merikangas KR, Rasmussen BK. Migraine comorbidity. In: Olesen J, Tfelt-Hansen P, Welch KM, editors. The headaches. 2nd edition. Philadelphia: Lippincott Williams and Wilkins; 2000. p. 235–40.
62. Scher AI, Bigal ME, Lipton RB. Comorbidity of migraine. Curr Opin Neurol 2005; 18(3):305–10.
63. Pietrobon D, Moskowitz MA. Pathophysiology of migraine. Annu Rev Physiol 2012;75:365–91.
64. Edvinsson L, Villalon CM, Maassenvandenbrink A. Basic mechanisms of migraine and its acute treatment. Pharmacol Ther 2012;136(3):319–33.
65. Pryse-Phillips WE, Dodick DW, Edmeads JG, et al. Guidelines for the nonpharmacologic management of migraine in clinical practice. Canadian Headache Society. CMAJ 1998;159(1):47–54.
66. Holland S, Silberstein SD, Freitag F, et al. Evidence-based guideline update: NSAIDs and other complementary treatments for episodic migraine prevention in adults: report of the Quality Standards Subcommittee of the American Academy of Neurology and the American Headache Society. Neurology 2012;78(17): 1346–53.
67. Dodick DW, Lipton RB, Ferrari MD, et al. Prioritizing treatment attributes and their impact on selecting an oral triptan: results from the TRIPSTAR Project. Curr Pain Headache Rep 2004;8(6):435–42.
68. Ferrari MD, Goadsby PJ, Roon KI, et al. Triptans (serotonin, 5-HT1B/1D agonists) in migraine: detailed results and methods of a meta-analysis of 53 trials. Cephalalgia 2002;22(8):633–58.
69. Savi L, Omboni S, Lisotto C, et al. Efficacy of frovatriptan in the acute treatment of menstrually related migraine: analysis of a double-blind, randomized, crossover, multicenter, Italian, comparative study versus rizatriptan. J Headache Pain 2011;12(6):609–15.
70. Silberstein SD, Holland S, Freitag F, et al. Evidence-based guideline update: pharmacologic treatment for episodic migraine prevention in adults: report of the Quality Standards Subcommittee of the American Academy of Neurology and the American Headache Society. Neurology 2012;78(17):1337–45.
71. MacGregor EA, Pawsey SP, Campbell JC, et al. Safety and tolerability of frovatriptan in the acute treatment of migraine and prevention of menstrual migraine: results of a new analysis of data from five previously published studies. Gend Med 2010;7(2):88–108.
72. US Headache Consortium. Evidence-based guidelines for migraine headache in the primary care setting: pharmacological management for prevention of migraine. American Academy of Neurology; 2000. Available at: http://www.aan.com/professionals/practice/pdfs/gl0090.pdf. Accessed October 2005.
73. Silberstein SD, Goadsby PJ, Lipton RB. Management of migraine: an algorithmic approach. Neurology 2000;55(9 Suppl 2):S46–52.
74. Loder E, Biondi D. General principles of migraine management: the changing role of prevention. Headache 2005;45(Suppl 1):S33–47.
75. Welch KM, Nagesh V, Aurora SK, et al. Periaqueductal gray matter dysfunction in migraine: cause or the burden of illness? Headache 2001;41(7):629–37.
76. Chronicle E, Mulleners W. Anticonvulsant drugs for migraine prophylaxis. Cochrane Database Syst Rev 2004;(3):CD003226.

77. Silberstein SD, Goadsby PJ. Migraine: preventive treatment. Cephalalgia 2002; 22(7):491–512.
78. Goadsby PJ. Advances in the understanding of headache. Br Med Bull 2005; 73–74:83–92.
79. Dahlof CG. Management of primary headaches: current and future aspects. In: Giamberardino MA, editor. Pain 2002- An updated review: refresher course. Seattle (WA): IASP Press; 2002. p. 85–112.
80. Leone M, Proietti Cecchini A, Franzini A, et al. From neuroimaging to patients' bench: what we have learnt from trigemino-autonomic pain syndromes. Neurol Sci 2012;33(Suppl 1):S99–102.
81. Holle D, Katsarava Z, Obermann M. The hypothalamus: specific or nonspecific role in the pathophysiology of trigeminal autonomic cephalalgias? Curr Pain Headache Rep 2011;15(2):101–7.
82. Leone M, Bussone G. Pathophysiology of trigeminal autonomic cephalalgias. Lancet Neurol 2009;8(8):755–64.
83. Manzoni GC, Terzano MG, Bono G, et al. Cluster headache—clinical findings in 180 patients. Cephalalgia 1983;3(1):21–30.
84. Fischera M, Marziniak M, Gralow I, et al. The incidence and prevalence of cluster headache: a meta-analysis of population-based studies. Cephalalgia 2008; 28(6):614–8.
85. Sjaastad O, Bakketeig LS. Cluster headache prevalence. Vaga study of headache epidemiology. Cephalalgia 2003;23(7):528–33.
86. Benoliel R, Sharav Y. Trigeminal autonomic cephalgias (TACs). In: Sharav Y, Benoliel R, editors. Orofacial pain and headache. Edinburgh (United Kingdom): Mosby Elsevier; 2008. p. 223–54.
87. van Vliet JA, Eekers PJ, Haan J, et al. Features involved in the diagnostic delay of cluster headache. J Neurol Neurosurg Psychiatry 2003;74(8):1123–5.
88. Manzoni GC, Micieli G, Granella F, et al. Cluster headache—course over ten years in 189 patients. Cephalalgia 1991;11(4):169–74.
89. Bahra A, Goadsby PJ. Diagnostic delays and mis-management in cluster headache. Acta Neurol Scand 2004;109(3):175–9.
90. Klapper JA, Klapper A, Voss T. The misdiagnosis of cluster headache: a nonclinic, population-based, Internet survey. Headache 2000;40(9):730–5.
91. Larner AJ. Trigeminal autonomic cephalalgias: frequency in a general neurology clinic setting. J Headache Pain 2008;9(5):325–6.
92. Van Alboom E, Louis P, Van Zandijcke M, et al. Diagnostic and therapeutic trajectory of cluster headache patients in Flanders. Acta Neurol Belg 2009; 109(1):10–7.
93. Cademartiri C, Torelli P, Cologno D, et al. Upper and lower cluster headache: clinical and pathogenetic observations in 608 patients. Headache 2002;42(7):630–7.
94. Bahra A, May A, Goadsby PJ. Cluster headache: a prospective clinical study with diagnostic implications. Neurology 2002;58(3):354–61.
95. Torelli P, Manzoni GC. Pain and behaviour in cluster headache. A prospective study and review of the literature. Funct Neurol 2003;18(4):205–10.
96. Russell D. Cluster headache: severity and temporal profiles of attacks and patient activity prior to and during attacks. Cephalalgia 1981;1(4):209–16.
97. Pfaffenrath V, Pollmann W, Ruther E, et al. Onset of nocturnal attacks of chronic cluster headache in relation to sleep stages. Acta Neurol Scand 1986;73(4):403–7.
98. Chervin RD, Zallek SN, Lin X, et al. Timing patterns of cluster headaches and association with symptoms of obstructive sleep apnea. Sleep Res Online 2000;3(3):107–12.

99. Schurks M, Diener HC. Cluster headache and lifestyle habits. Curr Pain Headache Rep 2008;12(2):115–21.
100. Torelli P, Cologno D, Cademartiri C, et al. Possible predictive factors in the evolution of episodic to chronic cluster headache. Headache 2000;40(10):798–808.
101. Blau JN, Engel HO. Premonitory and prodromal symptoms in cluster headache. Cephalalgia 1998;18(2):91–3 [discussion: 71–2].
102. Langedijk M, van der Naalt J, Luijckx GJ, et al. Cluster-like headache aura status. Headache 2005;45(1):80–1.
103. Drummond PD. Dissociation between pain and autonomic disturbances in cluster headache. Headache 1990;30(8):505–8.
104. Wheeler SD. Significance of migrainous features in cluster headache: divalproex responsiveness. Headache 1998;38(7):547–51.
105. Irimia P, Cittadini E, Paemeleire K, et al. Unilateral photophobia or phonophobia in migraine compared with trigeminal autonomic cephalalgias. Cephalalgia 2008;28(6):626–30.
106. Levy MJ, Matharu MS, Meeran K, et al. The clinical characteristics of headache in patients with pituitary tumours. Brain 2005;128(Pt 8):1921–30.
107. Manzoni GC. Cluster headache and lifestyle: remarks on a population of 374 male patients. Cephalalgia 1999;19(2):88–94.
108. Cittadini E, Matharu MS. Symptomatic trigeminal autonomic cephalalgias. Neurologist 2009;15(6):305–12.
109. Favier I, van Vliet JA, Roon KI, et al. Trigeminal autonomic cephalgias due to structural lesions: a review of 31 cases. Arch Neurol 2007;64(1):25–31.
110. Trucco M, Mainardi F, Maggioni F, et al. Chronic paroxysmal hemicrania, hemicrania continua and SUNCT syndrome in association with other pathologies: a review. Cephalalgia 2004;24(3):173–84.
111. Wilbrink LA, Ferrari MD, Kruit MC, et al. Neuroimaging in trigeminal autonomic cephalgias: when, how, and of what? Curr Opin Neurol 2009;22(3):247–53.
112. Goadsby PJ, Cittadini E, Cohen AS. Trigeminal autonomic cephalalgias: paroxysmal hemicrania, SUNCT/SUNA, and hemicrania continua. Semin Neurol 2010;30(2):186–91.
113. Dodick DW, Rozen TD, Goadsby PJ, et al. Cluster headache. Cephalalgia 2000;20(9):787–803.
114. Ashkenazi A, Schwedt T. Cluster headache—acute and prophylactic therapy. Headache 2011;51(2):272–86.
115. Rozen TD. Trigeminal autonomic cephalalgias. Neurol Clin 2009;27(2):537–56.
116. Rozen TD. High oxygen flow rates for cluster headache. Neurology 2004;63(3):593.
117. Antonaci F, Costa A, Candeloro E, et al. Single high-dose steroid treatment in episodic cluster headache. Cephalalgia 2005;25(4):290–5.
118. Benoliel R. Trigeminal autonomic cephalgias. B J Pain 2012;6(3):106–23.
119. Paemeleire K, Evers S, Goadsby PJ. Medication-overuse headache in patients with cluster headache. Curr Pain Headache Rep 2008;12(2):122–7.
120. Goadsby PJ, Cittadini E, Burns B, et al. Trigeminal autonomic cephalalgias: diagnostic and therapeutic developments. Curr Opin Neurol 2008;21(3):323–30.
121. Koopman JS, Dieleman JP, Huygen FJ, et al. Incidence of facial pain in the general population. Pain 2009;147(1–3):122–7.
122. Obermann M, Katsarava Z. Epidemiology of unilateral headaches. Expert Rev Neurother 2008;8(9):1313–20.

123. Sjaastad O, Bakketeig LS. The rare, unilateral headaches. Vaga study of head-ache epidemiology. J Headache Pain 2007;8(1):19–27.
124. Antonaci F, Sjaastad O. Chronic paroxysmal hemicrania (CPH): a review of the clinical manifestations. Headache 1989;29(10):648–56.
125. Boes CJ, Dodlck DW. Refining the clinical spectrum of chronic paroxysmal hem-icrania: a review of 74 patients. Headache 2002;42(8):699–708.
126. Kudrow DB, Kudrow L. Successful aspirin prophylaxis in a child with chronic paroxysmal hemicrania. Headache 1989;29(5):280–1.
127. Matharu MS, Goadsby PJ. Bilateral paroxysmal hemicrania or bilateral parox-ysmal cephalgia, another novel indomethacin-responsive primary headache syndrome? Cephalalgia 2005;25(2):79–81.
128. Boes CJ, Vincent M, Russell D. Chronic paroxysmal hemicrania. In: Olesen J, Goadsby PJ, Ramadan NM, et al, editors. The headaches. 3rd edition. Philadel-phia: Lippincott Williams & Wilkins; 2006. p. 815–22.
129. Sarlani E, Schwartz AH, Greenspan JD, et al. Chronic paroxysmal hemicrania: a case report and review of the literature. J Orofac Pain 2003;17(1):74–8.
130. Siow HC. Seasonal episodic paroxysmal hemicrania responding to cyclooxygenase-2 inhibitors. Cephalalgia 2004;24(5):414–5.
131. Sahota PK, Dexter JD. Sleep and headache syndromes: a clinical review. Head-ache 1990;30(2):80–4.
132. Benoliel R, Sharav Y. Paroxysmal hemicrania. Case studies and review of the literature. Oral Surg Oral Med Oral Pathol Oral Radiol Endod 1998;85(3):285–92.
133. Cittadini E, Matharu MS, Goadsby PJ. Paroxysmal hemicrania: a prospective clinical study of 31 cases. Brain 2008;131(Pt 4):1142–55.
134. Mariano da Silva H, Benevides-Luz I, Santos AC, et al. Chronic paroxysmal hemicrania as a manifestation of intracranial parotid gland carcinoma metas-tasis—a case report. Cephalalgia 2004;24(3):223–7.
135. Gatzonis S, Mitsikostas DD, Ilias A, et al. Two more secondary headaches mimicking chronic paroxysmal hemicrania. Is this the exception or the rule? Headache 1996;36(8):511–3.
136. Parcja J, Sjaastad O. Chronic paroxysmal hemicrania and hemicrania continua. Interval between indomethacin administration and response. Headache 1996; 36(1):20–3.
137. Sjaastad O, Antonaci F. Chronic paroxysmal hemicrania: a case report. Long-lasting remission in the chronic stage. Cephalalgia 1987;7(3):203–5.
138. Camarda C, Camarda R, Monastero R. Chronic paroxysmal hemicrania and hemicrania continua responding to topiramate: two case reports. Clin Neurol Neurosurg 2008;110(1):88–91.
139. Cohen AS, Goadsby PJ. Paroxysmal hemicrania responding to topiramate. J Neurol Neurosurg Psychiatry 2007;78(1):96–7.
140. Sjaastad O, Saunte C, Salvesen R, et al. Shortlasting unilateral neuralgiform headache attacks with conjunctival injection, tearing, sweating, and rhinorrhea. Cephalalgia 1989;9(2):147–56.
141. Sjaastad O, Kruszewski P. Trigeminal neuralgia and "SUNCT" syndrome: similar-ities and differences in the clinical pictures. An overview. Funct Neurol 1992; 7(2):103–7.
142. Pareja JA, Cuadrado ML. SUNCT syndrome: an update. Expert Opin Pharmac-other 2005;6(4):591–9.
143. Matharu MS, Cohen AS, Boes CJ, et al. Short-lasting unilateral neuralgiform headache with conjunctival injection and tearing syndrome: a review. Curr Pain Headache Rep 2003;7(4):308–18.

144. D'Andrea G, Granella F. SUNCT syndrome: the first case in childhood. Short-lasting unilateral neuralgiform headache attacks with conjunctival injection and tearing. Cephalalgia 2001;21(6):701–2.
145. Gantenbein AR, Goadsby PJ. Familial SUNCT. Cephalalgia 2005;25(6):457–9.
146. Cohen AS, Matharu MS, Goadsby PJ. Short-lasting unilateral neuralgiform headache attacks with conjunctival injection and tearing (SUNCT) or cranial autonomic features (SUNA)–a prospective clinical study of SUNCT and SUNA. Brain 2006;129(Pt 10):2746–60.
147. Pareja JA, Shen JM, Kruszewski P, et al. SUNCT syndrome: duration, frequency, and temporal distribution of attacks. Headache 1996;36(3):161–5.
148. Pareja JA, Caballero V, Sjaastad O. SUNCT syndrome. Statuslike pattern. Headache 1996;36(10):622–4.
149. Baldacci F, Nuti A, Lucetti C, et al. SUNA syndrome with seasonal pattern. Headache 2009;49(6):912–4.
150. Benoliel R, Sharav Y. Trigeminal neuralgia with lacrimation or SUNCT syndrome? Cephalalgia 1998;18(2):85–90.
151. Kruszewski P, Zhao JM, Shen JM, et al. SUNCT syndrome: forehead sweating pattern. Cephalalgia 1993;13(2):108–13.
152. Jacob S, Rajabally Y. Short-lasting unilateral neuralgiform headache with cranial autonomic symptoms (SUNA) following vertebral artery dissection. Cephalalgia 2007;27(3):283–5.
153. Jimenez Caballero PE, Portilla Cuenca JC, Casado Naranjo I. Short-lasting unilateral neuralgiform headache attacks with cranial autonomic symptoms (SUNA) secondary to epidermoid cyst in the right cerebellopontine angle successfully treated with surgery. J Headache Pain 2011;12(3):385–7.
154. Williams MH, Broadley SA. SUNCT and SUNA: clinical features and medical treatment. J Clin Neurosci 2008;15(5):526–34.
155. Pareja JA, Kruszewski P, Sjaastad O. SUNCT syndrome: trials of drugs and anesthetic blockades. Headache 1995;35(3):138–42.
156. Morales-Asin F, Espada F, Lopez-Obarrio LA, et al. A SUNCT case with response to surgical treatment. Cephalalgia 2000;20(1):67–8.
157. Benoliel R, Sharav Y. SUNCT syndrome: case report and literature review. Oral Surg Oral Med Oral Pathol Oral Radiol Endod 1998;85(2):158–61.
158. Pareja JA, Sjaastad O. SUNCT syndrome. A clinical review. Headache 1997;37(4):195–202.
159. Rossi P, Faroni J, Tassorelli C, et al. Diagnostic delay and suboptimal management in a referral population with hemicrania continua. Headache 2009;49(2):227–34.
160. Newman LC, Lipton RB, Solomon S. Hemicrania continua: ten new cases and a review of the literature. Neurology 1994;44(11):2111–4.
161. Newman LC, Lipton RB, Russell M, et al. Hemicrania continua: attacks may alternate sides [see comments]. Headache 1992;32(5):237–8.
162. Peres MF, Silberstein SD, Nahmias S, et al. Hemicrania continua is not that rare. Neurology 2001;57(6):948–51.
163. Peres MF, Siow HC, Rozen TD. Hemicrania continua with aura. Cephalalgia 2002;22(3):246–8.
164. Peres MF, Silberstein SD. Hemicrania continua responds to cyclooxygenase-2 inhibitors. Headache 2002;42(6):530–1.
165. Sjaastad O, Antonaci F. A piroxicam derivative partly effective in chronic paroxysmal hemicrania and hemicrania continua. Headache 1995;35(9):549–50.
166. Rasmussen BK. Epidemiology of headache. Cephalalgia 1995;15(1):45–68.

167. Lyngberg AC, Rasmussen BK, Jorgensen T, et al. Incidence of primary head-ache: a Danish epidemiologic follow-up study. Am J Epidemiol 2005;161(11): 1066–73.
168. Lyngberg AC, Rasmussen BK, Jorgensen T, et al. Has the prevalence of migraine and tension-type headache changed over a 12-year period? A Danish population survey. Eur J Epidemiol 2005;20(3):243–9.
169. Russell MB. Tension-type headache in 40-year-olds: a Danish population-based sample of 4000. J Headache Pain 2005;6(6):441–7.
170. Jensen R, Symon D. Epidemiology of tension-type headache. In: Olesen J, Goadsby PJ, Ramadan NM, et al, editors. The headaches. 3rd edition. Philadelphia: Lippincott Williams & Wilkins; 2006. p. 621–4.
171. Rasmussen BK, Jensen R, Olesen J. Impact of headache on sickness absence and utilisation of medical services: a Danish population study. J Epidemiol Community Health 1992;46(4):443–6.
172. Stovner LJ, Zwart JA, Hagen K, et al. Epidemiology of headache in Europe. Eur J Neurol 2006;13(4):333–45.
173. Ostergaard S, Russell MB, Bendtsen L, et al. Comparison of first degree relatives and spouses of people with chronic tension headache. BMJ 1997; 314(7087):1092–3.
174. Ulrich V, Gervil M, Olesen J. The relative influence of environment and genes in episodic tension-type headache. Neurology 2004;62(11):2065–9.
175. Iversen HK, Langemark M, Andersson PG, et al. Clinical characteristics of migraine and episodic tension-type headache in relation to old and new diagnostic criteria. Headache 1990;30(8):514–9.
176. Inan LE, Tulunay FC, Guvener A, et al. Characteristics of headache in migraine without aura and episodic tension-type headache in the Turkish population according to the IHS classification. Cephalalgia 1994;14(2):171–3.
177. Gobel H, Petersen-Braun M, Soyka D. The epidemiology of headache in Germany: a nationwide survey of a representative sample on the basis of the headache classification of the International Headache Society. Cephalalgia 1994; 14(2):97–106.
178. Rasmussen BK. Migraine and tension-type headache are separate disorders. Cephalalgia 1996;16(4):217–20 [discussion: 223].
179. Olesen J, Bousser MG, Diener HC, et al. The International classification of headache disorders, 2nd edition. Cephalalgia 2004;24(Suppl 1):24–150.
180. Couch JR. The long-term prognosis of tension-type headache. Curr Pain Headache Rep 2005;9(6):436–41.
181. Lipton RB, Cady RK, Stewart WF, et al. Diagnostic lessons from the spectrum study. Neurology 2002;58(9 Suppl 6):S27–31.
182. Lipton RB, Stewart WF, Cady R, et al. 2000 Wolfe Award. Sumatriptan for the range of headaches in migraine sufferers: results of the Spectrum Study. Headache 2000;40(10):783–91.
183. Ulrich V, Russell MB, Jensen R, et al. A comparison of tension-type headache in migraineurs and in non-migraineurs: a population-based study. Pain 1996; 67(2–3):501–6.
184. Koseoglu E, Nacar M, Talaslioglu A, et al. Epidemiological and clinical characteristics of migraine and tension type headache in 1146 females in Kayseri, Turkey. Cephalalgia 2003;23(5):381–8.
185. Bigal ME, Sheftell FD, Rapoport AM, et al. Chronic daily headache in a tertiary care population: correlation between the International Headache Society

diagnostic criteria and proposed revisions of criteria for chronic daily headache. Cephalalgia 2002;22(6):432–8.

186. Bendtsen L, Jensen R. Mirtazapine is effective in the prophylactic treatment of chronic tension-type headache. Neurology 2004;62(10):1706–11.

187. Manzoni GC, Granella F, Sandrini G, et al. Classification of chronic daily headache by International Headache Society criteria: limits and new proposals. Cephalalgia 1995;15(1):37–43.

188. Jensen R, Rasmussen BK. Muscular disorders in tension-type headache. Cephalalgia 1996;16(2):97–103.

189. Bendtsen L, Jensen R, Olesen J. Decreased pain detection and tolerance thresholds in chronic tension-type headache. Arch Neurol 1996;53(4):373–6.

190. Langemark M, Olesen J, Poulsen DL, et al. Clinical characterization of patients with chronic tension headache. Headache 1988;28(9):590–6.

191. de Filippis S, Salvatori E, Coloprisco G, et al. Headache and mood disorders. J Headache Pain 2005;6(4):250–3.

192. Bendtsen L, Fernandez-de-la-Penas C. The role of muscles in tension-type headache. Curr Pain Headache Rep 2011;15(6):451–8.

193. Bezov D, Ashina S, Jensen R, et al. Pain perception studies in tension-type headache. Headache 2011;51(2):262–71.

194. Kaniecki RG. Tension-type headache. Continuum 2012;18(4):823–34.

195. Mathew NT, Ashina M. Acute pharmacotherapy of tension-type headaches. In: Olesen J, Goadsby PJ, Ramadan NM, et al, editors. The headaches. 3rd edition. Philadelphia: Lippincott Williams & Wilkins; 2006. p. 727–33.

196. Steiner TJ, Lange R, Voelker M. Aspirin in episodic tension-type headache: placebo-controlled dose-ranging comparison with paracetamol. Cephalalgia 2003;23(1):59–66.

197. Brennum J, Kjeldsen M, Olesen J. The 5-HT1-like agonist sumatriptan has a significant effect in chronic tension-type headache. Cephalalgia 1992;12(6):375–9.

198. Cady RK, Gutterman D, Saiers JA, et al. Responsiveness of non-IHS migraine and tension-type headache to sumatriptan. Cephalalgia 1997;17(5):588–90.

199. Tomkins GE, Jackson JL, O'Malley PG, et al. Treatment of chronic headache with antidepressants: a meta-analysis. Am J Med 2001;111(1):54–63.

200. Fumal A, Schoenen J. Chronic tension-type headache. In: Goadsby PJ, Silberstein SD, Dodick D, editors. Chronic daily headache. Hamilton (Canada): BC Decker Inc; 2005. p. 57–64.

201. Stillman MJ. Pharmacotherapy of tension-type headaches. Curr Pain Headache Rep 2002;6(5):408–13.

202. Holroyd KA. Behavioral and psychologic aspects of the pathophysiology and management of tension-type headache. Curr Pain Headache Rep 2002;6(5):401–7.

203. Bogaards MC, ter Kuile MM. Treatment of recurrent tension headache: a meta-analytic review. Clin J Pain 1994;10(3):174–90.

204. Holroyd KA, O'Donnell FJ, Stensland M, et al. Management of chronic tension-type headache with tricyclic antidepressant medication, stress management therapy, and their combination: a randomized controlled trial. JAMA 2001; 285(17):2208–15.

205. Fernandez-de-Las-Penas C, Alonso-Blanco C, Cuadrado ML, et al. Are manual therapies effective in reducing pain from tension-type headache?: a systematic review. Clin J Pain 2006;22(3):278–85.

206. Magnusson T, Carlsson GE. A 2 1/2-year follow-up of changes in headache and mandibular dysfunction after stomatognathic treatment. J Prosthet Dent 1983; 49(3):398–402.
207. Vallon D, Ekberg E, Nilner M, et al. Occlusal adjustment in patients with cranio-mandibular disorders including headaches. A 3- and 6-month follow-up. Acta Odontol Scand 1995;53(1):55–9.

Topical Medications as Treatment of Neuropathic Orofacial Pain

Cibele Nasri-Heir, DDS, MSD, Junad Khan, BDS, MSD, MPH, DAAOP, Gary M. Heir, DMD*

KEYWORDS

- Neuropathic pain • Topical medication • Neuropathic orofacial pain • Orofacial pain

KEY POINTS

- Advantages of topical medications include
  - Avoidance of the gastrointestinal tract and hepatic first-pass biotransformation and metabolism
  - Delivery to a specific site
  - Control of absorption rate possible
  - Reduced systemic side effects
  - Improved compliance
- Understanding mechanisms of neuropathic orofacial pain (NOP), targets of treatment, and basic pharmacology and working with informed compounding pharmacists may result in significant benefit for patients.
- The clinical significance of this approach is the improvement of the quality of life for patients by providing a unique medication delivery system for NOP and other dental and extraoral conditions.
- The use of this route of administration has decreased or minimized side effects compared with other methods of administration and, therefore, is especially useful in medically compromised and elderly patients.
- Although not a replacement for systemic medications, these innovations, supported and improved by ongoing research, will augment the armamentarium of clinicians treating orofacial pain disorders.

I'm wondering how people manage with chronic pain? I don't want it to rule me. How can I rule it? I just feel desperate for suggestions. I really want to get control back. Pain has controlled my life for too long! Help!
—Anonymous online post to a pain support group

Department of Diagnostic Sciences, Center for Temporomandibular Disorders and Orofacial Pain, University of Medicine and Dentistry of New Jersey, 110 Bergen Street – Room D 860, Newark, NJ 07103, USA
* Corresponding author.
E-mail addresses: heirgm@umdnj.edu; heirgm@gmail.com

Dent Clin N Am 57 (2013) 541–553
http://dx.doi.org/10.1016/j.cden.2013.04.011
0011-8532/13/$ – see front matter © 2013 Published by Elsevier Inc.

dental.theclinics.com

OVERVIEW

Patients in pain routinely confront a dental clinician. Understanding pain mechanisms can aid in achieving an accurate diagnoses. Management of chronic orofacial pain often requires the assessment, diagnosis, and treatment of complex chronic pain disorders of nonodontogenic origin. An understanding of basic concepts of musculoskeletal, neuropathic, and neurovascular orofacial pain disorders is necessary to facilitate effective treatment. Appropriate management is the responsibility of clinicians and can have a direct impact on improving patients' quality of life.

Treatment of chronic pain and painful disorders involving the orofacial region often involves pharmacotherapeutic agents, which can be accompanied by unpleasant side effects. In addition, with the aging population, patients who are medically compromised or using multiple medications may have contraindications for commonly used orofacial pain medications, further challenging the treatment. This article discusses an alternate route of treatment.

INTRODUCTION

Pain is not a sensation but an individual experience. Like hunger or thirst, it is often difficult to define and varies from patient to patient. Understanding is in its infancy and there are increasingly complex challenges to understanding of pain. In the past, pain has been treated by blocking it with anesthetics or altering it with analgesics but the exact cause has not always been targeted. An increased understanding of the neurophysiology of pain, neurotransmitters, and their actions in pain transmission, however, has led to positive steps in selective pharmacotherapy that offer great hope for the future.

One chronic complex entity of orofacial pain is NOP disorders, which pose a significant challenge to dental practitioners. Patients often present with, or are referred for, the evaluation of pain complaints that are inappropriately thought to have dental etiologies. Many acute and chronic pain disorders not only mimic pain of odontogenic cause but also frequently are treated inappropriately with dental remedies. It is dental practitioners' responsibility to evaluate and diagnosis these disorders correctly to affect an appropriate course of treatment.

The International Association for the Study of Pain defines pain as "An unpleasant sensory and emotional experience associated with actual or potential tissue damage, or described in terms of such damage."[1] In many cases, such as acute pain, the cause is evident. A traumatic injury, dental infection, or intraoral lesion may be the source of noxious stimuli of primary afferent nociceptors that send the message of tissue damage to the central nervous system for processing and eventual perception as pain. Chronic pain disorders, such as neuralgias, chronic musculoskeletal disorders, and various forms of neurovascular pain, may produce equivalent pain but usually are not secondary to tissue damaging events. Neuropathic pain is defined as "pain caused by a lesion or dysfunction of the somatosensory nervous system." Lesions or diseases of the somatosensory system may occur peripherally or centrally.[2]

WHAT WE KNOW

The sensory system is a dynamic complex of neuronal tissue, driven and modified by a vast array of neurochemicals with myriad interactions, which in turn are acted on by endogenous and exogenous modifiers of its responsiveness. Multiple molecular and cellular mechanisms operate alone and in combination within the peripheral and central nervous systems to produce pain. These features offer the opportunity for unique compounds targeted at modifying specific pain mechanisms.

Pain process generally begins at the periphery, outside the brain and spinal cord. For more than 500 years, the Cartesian model has been the accepted concept of pain perception. In his 1664 *Treatise of Man*, René Descartes theorized that pain was a disturbance that traveled along fibers that reached the brain: "If the fire is close to the foot, the little particles of the fire which, as you know move very rapidly, are able to move the skin of the foot that they touch and thus, pulling the little thread. They immediately open the pores at the end of the thread just as by pulling one end of a rope instantly rings the bell hanging at the other end."[3] Logically, disruption of this signal was considered the ultimate treatment. Although often affective, this has not always been the case. Consider an event involving peripheral nerve damage or centrally mediated pain secondary to spinal cord or brainstem. Although Descartes was not incorrect, his theory was incomplete.

Nociceptors, when stimulated to threshold, indicate the presence of actual or potentially harmful stimuli. It is the brain, however, that interprets the signal as painful. Actual or potential tissue damage not only results in the direct stimulation of peripheral afferent nociceptors but also triggers a cascade of events that eventually leads to the perception of pain at the level of the somatosensory cortex. Noxious input is not perceived as painful until it reaches these higher centers.

Knowledge of the steps from the transformation of a noxious stimulus into a painful perception is necessary for understanding the manner in which these signals might be altered in a way to reduce or eliminate the eventual pain perception, perhaps using, in part, a Cartesian paradigm of disruption of the signal.

There are generally 4 separate steps along the path to pain perception. A nociceptor is a specialized nerve that fires in the presence of a noxious stimulus. Nociceptors do not fire as a result of typically non-noxious stimuli; a stronger, noxious input is necessary. The first step is a tissue-damaging or a potentially tissue-damaging stimulus that is capable of activating high threshold mechanical, chemical, or thermal receptors in the periphery. The change of any of these stimuli into the electrical impulse that initiates an action potential is referred to as transduction. Once any of these stimuli capable of transduction occurs, a second step occurs, that of transmission. The transduced impulse is transmitted along the primary afferent nociceptor, where it eventually synapses in the dorsal horn of the spinal cord, passing the stimulus on to numerous second-order neurons. Another step on the way to perception then occurs. Depending on the strength of the noxious stimulus and strength of synaptic connections of primary to second-order neurons, the signal is distributed to higher centers at the brainstem level for further processing and distribution. Before the signal moves on, however, a third step occurs at the dorsal horn. As the signal stimulates higher brainstem centers, it is attenuated by inhibitory pathways that send signals downstream reducing the strength of the pain signal, if not completely eliminating it. The combination of peripheral, large-diameter non-nociceptive fibers and thinner nociceptors brings mixed pain and nonpainful signals to the dorsal horn. Centrally released inhibitory neurochemicals travel downward along inhibitory pathways that serve to modulate these signals at their dorsal horn connections. Modulation is facilitated by both the endogenous pain inhibition system as well as the effects of the gate control mechanism.[1] Finally, the transduced, transmitted, and modulated noxious input arrives at the somatosensory cortex where it is perceived as pain.

These four physiologic steps of pain perception, described in an oversimplified manner—transduction, transmission, modulation and perception—offer three potential targets for pharmacotherapeutic management of chronic pain patients.

Physiologic Pain

The various physiologic phenomenon associated with pain perception are outlined. A closer look at each process illustrates the process and pathophysiologic conditions that may be associated with chronic neuropathic pain. Transduction may occur as a direct result of a noxious stimulation of a primary afferent nociceptor. The territory of the tissue injury is also flooded with inflammatory mediators that not only sensitize the stimulated receptors but also spread inflammation over a wider area lowering the firing threshold of adjacent nerves. Inflammatory molecules cause nociceptors to generate signals in the absence of any environmental input, referred to as primary hyperalgesia. This widened area of tenderness then can respond to non-noxious stimulation as if it were painful. Consider the pain of an insect bite that spreads over a wider field secondary to the spreading inflammation. This pain should resolve as the inflammation subsides and the injured area returns to normal.

Transmission of an action potential along the stimulated axon is the result of a barrage of depolarizing events along the cell membrane, mediated by sodium channels. All neurons have a balance point or resting potential during which no appreciable activity occurs. When stimulated, however, sodium ion channels embedded in the axonal membrane open and sodium ions enter the cell, resulting in the propagation of an action potential. This is the basis of the transmission of the signal along the primary afferent nerve. Therefore, a primary mechanism of normal pain transmission depends on the normal activity of sodium channels to open only in the presence of a transduced signal secondary to a noxious stimulus. After a physiologic action potential, the cell briefly hyperpolarizes and returns to the normal resting state.

As the transduced and transmitted action potential reaches the central nervous system at the spinal cord dorsal horn, it releases excitatory amino acids, such as glutamate, that cross the synaptic cleft to pass the signal along to the second-order neurons. This process is facilitated by the influx of calcium. As the action potential reaches the second-order connection, the influx of calcium initiates the migrations of neurotransmitter-filled vesicles to the cell's presynaptic membrane, releasing its contents into the synaptic cleft, a process referred to as exocytosis, thereby allowing the signal to make the second-order connection. These may be nociceptive second-order neurons, wide dynamic range neurons, or mechanoreceptors. At this point in the dorsal horn, there are complex interactions that require a brief explanation.

Descartes was not aware that nerve fibers are not merely simple threads that carried a signal. Nerves consist of bundles of various types of neurons carrying many different types of signals. The stimulation of non-nociceptive fibers, such as large, heavily myelinated A beta fibers, normally results in non-noxious signals, such as light touch. Smaller A delta and C fibers carry noxious signals. The raw data carried by these differing fibers arrive at the dorsal horn, where they may cancel each other or, if one is stronger than the other, bring a perception of pain or touch. This is the essence of the gate control theory described by Melzack and Wall.[1] As the input arrives at the second-order neurons, the signal (not yet perceived as pain) is either facilitated or inhibited by the release of inhibitory neuropeptides that act on pain transmission. These inhibitory neurochemicals include serotonin and γ-aminobutyric acid (GABA). As the peripheral signal arrives, the gate control mechanism allows it to pass through as noxious or non-noxious, and the down-regulating system of the higher centers either inhibit or facilitate its further journey where it is perceived at step 4, perception. This scenario is beyond simplistic and is meant to illustrate 4 potential targets of pharmacotherapy for chronic neuropathic pain patients.

WHAT CAN GO WRONG?

Transduction occurs after noxious stimulation of a nociceptor. Activation of the nociceptors should usually end immediately on withdrawal of the noxious stimulus. Nociceptors are categorized as thinly myelinated, fast-conducting A delta fibers typically associated with fast sharp pain, and the slow conducting C fibers typically associated with more diffuse, chronic pain often associated with aching or burning. In the presence of inflammation, the firing threshold of nociceptors decreases until the inflammation resolves. Nociceptors fire in the absence of a noxious input. The result is allodynia (pain to a nonpainful stimulus) and hyperalgesia (an increased pain response to a typically painful stimulus). Another phenomenon may occur in the presence of peripheral damage. A-beta fibers that typically do not carry noxious signals convert to nociceptors, thereby creating an environment where light touch becomes painful.[4]

Along with pleomorphic changes of A-beta fibers, for reasons currently under investigation, a small percentage of patients reports continuous discomfort consistent with continuous activation of C fibers, such as ongoing hyperalgesia and allodynia. Imagine the pain of sunburn that lasts long after the skin has healed. Problems that may occur in the transmission of action potentials may arise because of damage to the primary afferent nociceptors. The model for this form of neuropathic pain is herpes zoster, or shingles, resulting in postherpetic neuralgia (PHN) secondary to damage caused by the herpes virus as it travels along the nerve. With PHN, pain may be produced by injured receptors, injured primary afferent neurons, changes at the dorsal root ganglia where the afferent cell bodies are located, or at the dorsal horn of the spinal cord. The pathophysiology of PHN is the stimulation of an inflammatory process along the affected nerves, offering at least 3 targets for treatment (ie, sensitization of peripheral receptors, damage to afferent fibers, and changes of spinal neurons).

Other examples of direct or indirect neuronal injury that might occur include needle stick injuries or as might occur during the placement of dental implants. A nerve may be directly traumatized by mechanical means during dental procedures or may indirectly be altered in its physiologic function due to local inflammation secondary to an operative procedure. At the site of trauma, sodium channels are up-regulated from the soma of the cell, which resides in the dorsal root ganglia. They overpopulate the membrane of the axon at the site of injury. The potentially robust representation of sodium channels at the site of trauma makes the cell membrane unstable causing the potential for ectopic discharge of the injured neuron producing action potentials, which report pain to the brain as if it had originated from the target of the injured nerve rather than the site of injury.

Another phenomenon that occurs at the site of neuronal trauma is the up-regulation of α-adrenergic receptors that are sensitive to circulating noradrenaline. These adrenergic receptors also sensitize the injured nerve to these catecholamines that are released during sympathetic nervous system activity, also with potential of generating action potentials. Finally, when nerve tissue is traumatized, it has a tendency to release neuropeptides, such as nerve growth factor, in attempts to repair the damage. Their release from an injured axon also serve to sensitize neighboring noninjured axons in the surrounding territory causing the spread of the dysfunctional noxious input.

Facilitation and inhibition of pain occurs at the dorsal horn input of afferent nociceptors and A beta fibers. Two phenomena may occur among many at this level of modulation. There may be a decrease of inhibitory neuropeptides, resulting in a lack of pain inhibition, and, in the presence of chronic pain, synaptic connections may strengthen as a result of the opening of additional receptors on the second-order neurons, known as *N*-methyl-D-aspartate (NMDA) receptors, further strengthening the synaptic

connections. Diminished down-regulating inhibition and strengthening of synaptic connections tend to amplify any noxious input. In addition, chronic pain input may result in
the opening of otherwise dormant intersegmental neuronal pathways within the spinal
cord that sensitizes and strengthens second-order connections, resulting in pain over a
wider area; the phenomenon is referred to as secondary hyperalgesia, and widening of
the receptive field of pain to noninjured areas. This phenomenon is due to spreading
noxious input to adjacent areas in the spinal cord due to release of central neuropeptides, such as glutamate, substance P, and opening of NMDA channels.

When these misinterpreted signals eventually arrive at the somatosensory cortex,
they are often perceived as different from or stronger than the actual stimulus that provoked them. These sensorial distortions result in allodynia or hyperalgesia and often
result in changes in brain function that have been documented in functional MRI
studies (**Fig. 1**).[5,6]

WHAT TO DO?

Commonly used medications for treatment of neuropathic pain include

- Analgesics
- Antidepressants
- Antihypertensives (eg, β-adrenergic antagonists and calcium channel antagonists)
- Antiepileptic drugs
- Adjunctive neuropathic pain medications
- Triptans and ergot derivatives
- Antianxiety agents
- Muscle relaxants
- Corticosteroids
- Antihistamines
- Local anesthetics

These drugs are used both therapeutically and, in some instances, prophylactically,
based on the particular pain syndrome or side effect being managed or anticipated.

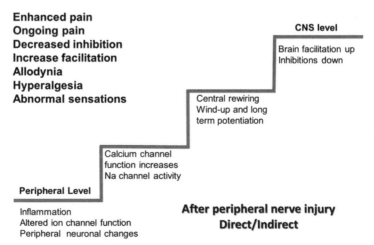

Fig. 1. Events follow neuronal trauma, leading to neuropathic pain and central sensitization. (*Courtesy of* Dr Gary Heir, Newark, New Jersey.)

Their use may be contraindicated in some cases or may result in intolerable side effects.

TOPICAL MEDICATIONS

Attempts to provide relief for those with chronic pain have included surgical and pharmacologic strategies directed at the symptom of pain, often with only limited success. One reason for this failure may be that not all potential targets for treatment are considered. Given that some patients cannot tolerate drug interactions or side effects of the medications (listed previously), an alternative to oral, rectal, or parenteral administration is a topical route.

The use of medications incorporated into topical gels has been used since the mid-1990s with the patent of a topical formulation for local delivery of a pharmaceutically active agents by E.G. Roentsch. Since the original patent in 1995, topical medications have been prescribed as creams, lotions, gels, ointment, liquid, powder, and sprays and formulated for intraoral use as troches, lollipops, and mouth rinses. Topical medications are applied directly to the painful or affected site where they exert their pharmacologic actions. Site of application include local peripheral tissues with the goal of affecting a change or pharmacologic action on peripheral receptors. By reducing the noxious traffic conducted along a pathophysiologic distribution of pain (ie, by reducing the noise on the system), the central pain process is diminished.

Neuropathic pain begins with an entry into the central nervous system via the peripheral system. Pain from the periphery may be considered either inflammatory or neuropathic. Continuous noxious input can lead to central sensitization and neuropathic pain syndromes. Central nervous system changes associated with central sensitization include hyperactivity of pain-transmission pathways, an increase in the number of receptors that respond to the neurotransmitters released by nociceptors, reorganization of central nociceptive connections, and loss of inhibitory function.[7] Ongoing pain leads to sensitization and exacerbates and prolongs discomfort. Blocking or reducing the peripheral input can result in the reduction or elimination of the effect.

Topical preparations that treat peripheral inflammation are in common use (ie, topical salicylates and diclofenac). There is also evidence of peripheral opioid receptors that may be affected by the local administration of opioids.[8] Other studies have demonstrated the presence of α-adrenergic receptors in the periphery after peripheral injury.[9] Many studies show the efficacy of topical in the facial region. They include the use of gabapentin, amethocaine, clonazepam, and capsacian for the treatment of various orofacial conditions, including trigeminal neuralgia, PHN, and itch related to neuropathy.[10–19]

Topicals include the ease of administration and the fact that this may be the route of choice for medically compromised patients. Optimized drug concentration occurs at the site of pain with minimal, if any, systemic uptake. Therefore, there is no need to titrate to affective levels. There are no drug interactions and negligible side effects other than an occasional local allergy or a rash.

Before continuing this discussion, a clear distinction between topical and transdermal medications is necessary. As discussed previously, a topical medication applied directly to the painful or affected area is absorbed at the selected site. The application is typically to local peripheral tissues, both extraorally and intraorally, where it results in a local effect with usually no systemic uptake. In contrast, transdermal medications require a clinically effective serum concentration for their efficacy, and their site of actions is remote from the site of administration. An example of a topical medication is a lidocaine patch with local affects compared with a transdermal nicotine patch with systemic distribution of the medication (**Table 1**).

A discussion has already been offered that identifies normal or physiologic pain as moving from the peripheral noxious stimulus to eventual perception with four distinct stops along the way that might influence the potential pain signals in a negative manner (ie, transduction, transmission, modulation, and perception). A partial list of systemic medications is suggested. Most of these medications can be prepared as topical medications.

MECHANISMS

Medications that are already Food and Drug Administration (FDA) approved are incorporated into a biologically inert vehicle through a milling process whereby the medications are reduced to a molecular level. Depending on the desired speed and depth of penetration, a soybean organogel or alcohol-based media may be used. The most commonly used transdermal/topical drug delivery system is pluronic lecithin organogel. Pluronic lecithin organogel is an opaque, yellow preparation composed of isopropyl palmitate, soy lecithin, water, and a pluronic surfactant. As suggested, by its name, it consists of an oil phase of lecithin dissolved in isopropyl palmitate and an aqueous phase of the surfactant.[20] Other anhydrous gel bases comprise propylene glycol, ethoxydiglycol, and glycerin in varying percentages. Ratios of propylene glycol:ethoxydiglycol determine depth of penetration. Increased concentrations of ethoxydiglycol result in more shallow penetration, which is, for example, advantageous in targeting nerve endings in the dermal layer.

A discussion of the pharmacology of compounding of topical medication is not included in this review; however, the result of proper compounding techniques results in the formation of micelles, small structures that encapsulate the molecules of medication. Micelles are small, spherical structures composed of a few dozen to thousands of molecules that attract one another to reduce surface tension within a membrane. The head of the molecule is hydrophilic (water soluble). The interior is hydrophobic (lipid soluble). Water cannot penetrate into the core of the aggregate sphere. Both hydrophilic and hydrophobic, these micelles penetrate both the lipid and water based layers of the skin or mucosa to deliver the topical medications after diffusion.

The efficacy of the topical preparation depends on proper compounding, the accuracy of the diagnosis, and the selection of the appropriate target for the medications. It must reach the target via appropriate penetration depth and speed of penetration to be effective. For example, if a patient has a superficial neuropathic pain disorder

Table 1 Topical vs Transdermal		
	Topical	**Transdermal**
Applications site	Applied directly to painful site	Distant from region or site of action
Site of activity	Peripherally (soft tissue)	Systemically
Serum drug concentrations	Insignificant	Expected
Systemic side effects	No	Yes
Titration necessary	No	Yes
Drug interactions	No	Yes

Courtesy of Dr Gary Heir, Newark, New Jersey.

exhibiting ectopic action potentials (excessive sodium channel sensitivity) and an increased sense of spreading burning discomfort with emotional stress (stimulation of α-adrenergic receptors), a topical preparation, including a sodium channel stabilizer and adrenergic receptor agonist, might be considered appropriate. If the preparation achieves a depth of penetration that does not reach the affected innervation, it fails to impart any benefit. In contrast, topical preparations that penetrate too quickly may have a brief therapeutic effect, followed by the report that the medication may have helped but not for long. The preparation may have passed through the level of the target too rapidly. It was effective but not at the optimal location for a long-enough period. Penetration speed and depth can be adjusted by a skilled compounding pharmacist.

Diffusion through the skin or mucosa involves what is referred to as a partition effect. For example, to deliver topical medications through the skin, the preparation must pass though first the stratum corneum, the epidermis, and eventually the dermis. At each interface, a hydrophilic or lipophilic barrier to drug diffusion is encountered, which delays the absorption of the medication until adequate levels eventually pass through.

In a retrospective study performed at the Center for Temporomandibular Disorders and Orofacial Pain, University of Medicine and Dentistry of New Jersey, 39 patients with neuropathic pain diagnosed with deafferentation pain, traumatic neuroma, or traumatic trigeminal neuralgia were subdivided in 3 categories. One group was treated only with a topical preparation specific for neuropathic pain; another group received conventional systemic medications; and the third group received combined topical and systemic medications.[21] The topical medication was a pluronic lecithin organogel that included carbamazepine 4%, lidocaine 1%, ketoprofen 4%, ketamine 4%, and gabapentin 4%. Systemic medications included carbamazepine, oxcarbamazepine, amitriptyline, or nortriptyline. Topical medications were applied by patients up to 4 times per day. Systemic medications were prescribed per standard pharmaceutical regimens.

Before and after the study, the patients self-reported their symptoms using a visual analog scale. All 3 groups demonstrated improvement (**Table 2**); however, the onset of relief for the topical-only group began at 3 weeks whereas the other 2 groups required an additional 1 to 2.5 weeks for maximum benefit.

From the results of this pilot study, it was concluded that topical medications used alone or in combination with systemic medications were highly effective in providing rapid pain relief compared with systemic medications alone. This pilot study became the basis for further studies to evaluate the use of topical medications in the treatment of orofacial neuropathic pain conditions.

A second study endeavored to demonstrate the use of topical medications as effective treatment of NOP in a prospective animal study.[22] For this study, an infraorbital chronic constrictive injury was surgically induced in rats. Once they exhibited chronic

Table 2
Topical, systemic and systemic–topical comparison

	Starting VAS	After Treatment VAS	Weeks Necessary for Maximum Benefit
Combined therapy	7.5 ± 0.403	3.6	5.5
Systemic medications only	8.6 ± 0.611	5.1	4
Topical medications only	6.1 ± 0.716	3.6	3

pain behavior, they were divided into groups treated with a topical vehicle with no medication and topical medications limited to pregabalin at 5% and at 10% and diclofenac at 5%. The goal of the study was to induce NOP in rats, assess pain behavior after topical application of pregabalin and/or diclofenac, and assess side effects of topical pregabalin and/or diclofenac in a rat model of neuropathic pain. At the conclusion of the study, serum concentrations of pregabalin and diclofenac were measured. Not only did the test animals treated with 10% pregabalin show a significant return to normal behavior signifying pain reduction but also studies performed testing endurance and coordination found no impairment in this group. Blood levels of the medications were insignificant.

The clinical application and importance of the findings of the animal study are the potential to improve quality of life of medically compromised or drug-sensitive individuals with a novel approach to drug and administration that has been shown to have a decrease in the side effects compared with other methods of administration.

WHAT CAN WE DO NOW?

It must be stressed that although there are preparations and formulations of topical medications routinely used, there is little standardization at this time. In addition, patients often have specific needs and custom-compounded topical preparations can be altered as necessary.

A brief discussion of NOP described various mechanisms and targets for treatment. Medications that can be manipulated into a topical formulation include

- Reduce peripheral inflammation
  - Nonsteroidal anti-inflammatory
- Abnormal sodium channel and α-adrenergic receptor expression along primary afferent nociceptors
  - Tricyclic antidepressants
  - Local and topical anesthetics
  - Some antiepileptic drugs
- Increased glutamate receptor activity
  - NMDA antagonists
  - AMPA antagonist
- Altered GABA inhibition
  - GABAergic agents
  - Anticonvulsants
  - Baclofen
- Calcium influx
  - Gabapentin
  - Pregablin

These medications may not always be effective and, if effective, may result in minimal improvement. Clinical experiences and recent studies conducted at the Center for Temporomandibular Disorders and Orofacial Pain at the New Jersey Dental School find that a positive affect occurs in approximately 75% of patients, with a range of improvement of 30% to 75%, although some patients achieve greater improvement. In cases of limited success, supplementation with systemic medication may be necessary but at much lower doses when combined with topicals.

Table 3 offers examples of ingredients of topical neuropathic medicates. Not all are used simultaneously and the use of clonidine and capsaicin is limited to selected cases.

Table 3
Some ingredients of topical neuropathic medications

	Commercially Available	Compounded
Examples	Capsaicin lidocaine/prilocaine topical 1 to 2.5 weeks Lidocaine patch Diclofenac 3%	Ketamine 5% Lidocaine 4% Ketoprofen 5%–10% Gabapentin 6% Carbamazapine 4% Clonidine 0.2%–0.4% Capsaicin .025% Pregalin 5%–10%
Considerations	Consistency of preparation Established safety and efficacy (FDA)	Potential variability of preparation Lack of controlled trials

Examples of other useful compounds in daily dental practice for treatment of painful conditions:

Intraoral ulcers
  Misoprostol
- Prostaglandin E2–misoprostol
- Action
  - Re-epithelialization, decreases pain and inflammation
  - Heals intraoral lesions within 24 hours
  - Stimulates bone growth
- Oral rinses, orabase, and sprays
  - Stimulate collagen repair
  - Reduce peripheral sensitization
- Indications
  - Oral stomatitis
  - Nonsteroidal anti-inflammatory drug–induced, viral-induced, chemotherapy-induced, or radiation-induced ulcers

Fever sores
  Deoxy D-glucose 0.2%
- Natural sugar, reverse isomer of glucose
- Actions
  - Antiviral
  - Similar to acyclovir
- Indications
  - Apthous ulcers
  - Herpes simplex virus
- Lip balms and oral rinses
- Transdermal
- Troche
- May be combined with topical anesthetic

Musculoskeletal pain
  Guaifenesin 10%
  - Topical cream made with Lipoderm
  Phenoxybenzamine (with caution) 0.5%–1.0%

Other possible dental compounds include

- Dry socket mixtures

- Root canal pastes
- Plaque removal solutions
- Plaque disclosure solution
- Reformulations of discontinued medications and preparations

SUMMARY

Advantages of topical medications include

- Avoidance of the gastrointestinal tract and hepatic first-pass biotransformation and metabolism
- Delivered to a specific site
- Control of absorption rate possible
- Time release
- Constant dosing
- Reduced systemic side effects
- Improved compliance

Understanding mechanisms of NOP, targets of treatment, and basic pharmacology and working with informed compounding pharmacists may result in significant benefit for patients. The clinical significance of this approach is the improvement of the quality of life for patients by providing a unique medication delivery system for NOP and other dental and extraoral conditions. The use of this route of administration has decreased or minimal side effects compared with other methods of administration and, therefore, is especially useful in medically compromised and elderly patients. Although not a replacement for systemic medications, these innovations, supported and improved by ongoing research, will augment the armamentarium of clinicians treating orofacial pain disorders.

REFERENCES

1. Melzack R, Wall PD. Pain mechanisms: a new theory. Science 1965;150(3699): 971–9.
2. Merskey H, Bogduk N. Classification of chronic pain: descriptions of chronic pain syndromes and definition of pain terms. 2nd edition. Seattle (WA): IASP; 1994.
3. Descartes R. Treatise of man. Harvard monographs in the history of science. Cambridge (United Kingdom): Harvard University Press; 1972.
4. Eliav E, Benoliel R, Tal M. Inflammation with no axonal damage of the rat saphenous nerve trunk induces ectopic discharge and mechanosensitivity in myelinated axons. Neurosci Lett 2001;311(1):49–52.
5. Borsook D, DaSilva AF, Ploghaus A, et al. Specific and somatotopic functional magnetic resonance imaging activation in the trigeminal ganglion by brush and noxious heat. J Neurosci 2003;23(21):7897–903.
6. Arthurs OJ, Boniface SJ. What aspect of the fMRI BOLD signal best reflects the underlying electrophysiology in human somatosensory cortex? Clin Neurophysiol 2003;114(7):1203–9.
7. Dubner R. Hyperalgesia and central nervous system plasticity in advances in temporomandibular disorders and orofacial pain. In: Fricton J, Dubner R, editors. New York: Raven Press; 1995. p. 67–71.
8. Joris JL, Dubner R, Hargreaves KM. Opioid analgesia at peripheral sites - a target for opioids released during stress and inflammation. Anesth Analg 1987; 66(12):1277–81.

9. Sato J, Perl ER. Adrenergic excitation of cutaneous pain receptors induced by peripheral nerve injury. Science 1991;251(5001):1608–10.

10. Amos K, Yeoh SC, Farah CS. Combined topical and systemic clonazepam therapy for the management of burning mouth syndrome: a retrospective pilot study. J Orofac Pain 2011;25(2):125–30.

11. Formaker BK, Mott AE, Frank ME. The effects of topical anesthesia on oral burning in burning mouth syndrome. Ann N Y Acad Sci 1998;855:776–80.

12. Hirsch AR, Ziad A, Kim AY, et al. Pilot study: alleviation of pain in burning mouth syndrome with topical sucralose. Headache 2011;51(3):444–6.

13. Kho HS, Lee JS, Lee EJ, et al. The effects of parafunctional habit control and topical lubricant on discomforts associated with burning mouth syndrome (BMS). Arch Gerontol Geriatr 2010;51(1):95–9.

14. Rodriguez de Rivera Campillo E, Lopez-Lopez J, Chimenos-Kustner E. Response to topical clonazepam in patients with burning mouth syndrome: a clinical study. Bull Group Int Rech Sci Stomatol Odontol 2010;49(1):19–29.

15. Padilla M, Clark GT, Merrill RL. Topical medications for orofacial neuropathic pain: a review. J Am Dent Assoc 2000;131(2):184–95.

16. Epstein JB, Marcoe JH. Topical application of capsaicin for treatment of oral neuropathic pain and trigeminal neuralgia. Oral Surg Oral Med Oral Pathol 1994;77(2):135–40.

17. Brill S, Ben-Abraham R, Goor-Aryeh I. Topical ophthalmic amethocaine alleviates trigeminal neuralgia pain. Local Reg Anesth 2010;3:155–7.

18. Sayanlar J, Guleyupoglu N, Portenoy R, et al. Trigeminal postherpetic neuralgia responsive to treatment with capsaicin 8% topical patch: a case report. J Headache Pain 2012;13(7):587–9.

19. Nakamizo S, Miyachi Y, Kabashima K. Treatment of neuropathic itch possibly due to trigeminal trophic syndrome with 0.1% topical tacrolimus and gabapentin. Acta Derm Venereol 2010;90(6):654–5.

20. Murdan S. Organogels in drug delivery. Expert Opin Drug Deliv 2005;2(3): 489–505.

21. Heir G, Karolchek S, Kalladka M, et al. Use of topical medication in orofacial neuropathic pain: a retrospective study. Oral Surg Oral Med Oral Pathol Oral Radiol Endod 2008;105(4):466–9.

22. Plaza-Villegas F, Heir G, Markman S, et al. Topical pregabalin and diclofenac for the treatment of neuropathic orofacial pain in rats. Oral Surg Oral Med Oral Pathol Oral Radiol 2012;114(4):449–56.

Index

Note: Page numbers of article titles are in **boldface** type.

Dent Clin N Am 57 (2013) 555–560
http://dx.doi.org/10.1016/S0011-8532(13)00046-3
0011-8532/13/$ – see front matter © 2013 Elsevier Inc. All rights reserved.

dental.theclinics.com

Moving?

Make sure your subscription moves with you!

To notify us of your new address, find your **Clinics Account Number** (located on your mailing label above your name), and contact customer service at:

Email: journalscustomerservice-usa@elsevier.com

800-654-2452 (subscribers in the U.S. & Canada)
314-447-8871 (subscribers outside of the U.S. & Canada)

Fax number: 314-447-8029

Elsevier Health Sciences Division
Subscription Customer Service
3251 Riverport Lane
Maryland Heights, MO 63043

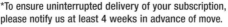

ELSEVIER